the Healing
Secrets of Food

the Healing Secrets of Food

A Practical Guide for Nourishing Body, Mind, and Soul

DEBORAH KESTEN

FOREWORD BY DEAN ORNISH, M.D.

New World Library
14 Pamaron Way
Novato, California 94949

New World Library
14 Pamaron Way
Novato, California 94949

Grateful acknowledgment is made to the following for permission to
use previously published material: From "Flirtation," by Rita Dove from
Museum, Carnegie-Mellon University Press. Copyright © 1983 by Rita
Dove. Reprinted by permission of the author. All rights reserved. From
The Illuminated Rumi by Coleman Barks and Michael Green. Copyright
© 1997 by Coleman Barks and Michael Green. Used by permission of
Broadway Books, a division of Random House, Inc.

Library of Congress Cataloging-in-Publication Data
Kesten, Deborah
  The healing secrets of food : a practical guide for nourishing body,
mind, and soul / Deborah Kesten.
      p.   cm.
Includes bibliographical references and index.
  ISBN 1-57731-188-4
1. Nutrition. 2. Food habits. 3. Dinners and dining — Psychological
aspects. 4. Dinners and dining — Social aspects. I. Title.
RA784 .K3995 2001
613.2 — dc21   2001002232

First Printing, August 2001
ISBN 1-57731-188-4
Printed in Canada on acid-free paper
Distributed to the trade by Publishers Group West

10 9 8 7 6 5 4 3

For my husband, Larry,
whose heart holds the healing secrets...and more,
with infinite love and gratitude.

❧

Contents

In order to understand how healing happens, in the twenty-first century we shall look not only at our atoms and molecules but at consciousness as well.
In so doing, we shall reinvent medicine, adding ancient wisdom to modern science.

—Larry Dossey, M.D.

foreword

꒳

Since nutritional science was born in the 1840s, when scientists first began to understand the complex structure of carbohydrates, proteins, fats, and minerals, the idea that what we eat has a powerful influence on healing or harming us has had a strong influence on American society. Today most of us take for granted that what we eat plays an important role in our health and well-being.

An increasing number of studies has shown that a low-fat, whole-foods, plant-based diet often provides a double benefit. These foods are low in disease-causing substances such as cholesterol, saturated fat, and oxidants while being rich in disease-fighting constituents such as antioxidants, fiber, phytochemicals, bioflavonoids, carotenoids, and so on. Scientists are finally beginning to document the literally thousands of food components with anti–heart disease, anticancer, and even antiaging properties. The more we look, the more we find to help explain why what we eat is so important.

In *The Healing Secrets of Food*, Deborah Kesten takes this research to the next level, describing a new model of nutrition that merges ancient food wisdom with state-of-the-art science. Her intriguing, well-researched message is that food influences all aspects of our health. She addresses not only the physical dimensions of nutrition but also the psychosocial, emotional, and spiritual dimensions of what and how we eat.

Many people are aware that our emotions affect what we eat. For example, people often overeat or gorge on fatty foods when they are feeling tired, depressed, or lonely. Deborah describes how many traditions take this concept even further: different types of food may influence our emotions, not just reflect our emotions.

She also holds that how we prepare our food and the way we eat it may also influence how different foods affect our emotional states.

Dr. Dennis Burkitt once wrote, "Not everything that counts can be counted." Science, including nutritional science, tends to focus on what can be measured, but not everything that is meaningful is measurable. Sometimes the most important aspects of our lives are those most difficult to quantify. It is rare to find someone who can skillfully walk the tightrope between scientifically proven nutritional concepts and those that are more difficult to prove yet are often even more meaningful. In *The Healing Secrets of Food*, Deborah Kesten has done just that. She coined the term *integrative nutrition* to describe her total approach to food and eating, beyond nutrition to true nourishment, that which feeds our body and soul.

As she writes, "While the intention of nutritional science is to provide objective truth about food (such as the influence of various nutrients on our physical health), it does not flavor food and meals with meaning. During the twentieth century, not only have we processed out the initial, inherent integrity of our food, we have also tossed aside the ageless, invisible, meaningful nourishment that food provides not only to our body but also to our emotional, spiritual, and social well-being." Along with applying key, objective, science-based nutritional concepts, the healing secrets presented in this book include bringing personalized, subjective depth and substance to the concept of nutritional health. Deborah's personal stories and new nutrition strategies may help transform your relationship to food.

Dean Ornish, M.D.
Founder, president, and director, Preventive Medicine
Research Institute Clinical Professor of Medicine,
School of Medicine, University of California, San Francisco

PART ONE

Nourishing Body, Mind, and Soul

A Broader View: Integrative Nutrition

I t's unfortunate that the healing powers of food have been kept a secret for so long. Although there's been no conscious conspiracy, no health-care cover-up, and no intentional oversight, most of us are in the dark about the many ways in which food heals us.

We're paying a big price for our ignorance: like a silent thief, it's robbing us of our health — physically, emotionally, spiritually, and socially. I wrote this book so that the secrets inherent in food won't remain secrets. After all, they're too important to all of us. Every aspect of our lives — even of the world and the planet — can potentially be healed by them.

In *The Healing Secrets of Food,* I am inviting you to join me on a journey that charts new nutritional territory. With my groundbreaking, cutting-edge strategies, I'll take you to a place that nourishes you each time you eat. To help you successfully navigate your way through this new terrain, beginning with your very next meal, I'll show you how to: eat to prevent or reverse physical ailments, experience the food-mood connection, reunite with the spiritual meaning of food, and reclaim your "social nutrition" heritage. With these health-enhancing tools at your table, you'll be empowered to unlock your health potential and to achieve your personal nutrition and wellness goals.

If you've already glanced at the table of contents, you've seen what I've listed as the healing secrets of food: the links among food, health, and socializing, feelings, mindfulness, appreciation, connection, and optimal food. You may be wondering, What's so secret about these? After all, aren't most of us familiar with these words? Don't we know what they mean?

But have you ever considered these concepts in terms of food? Most of us haven't. Do you know that eating with mindfulness and appreciation, for example, may enhance your health? Most of us don't. These healing secrets have been buried, ignored, diminished, and overlooked as the powerful healing tools they are. You can change this trend and reap the endless benefits of food — if you're willing to blaze a new nutrition trail.

A "New View": The Four Facets of Food

In *Ageless Body, Timeless Mind,* Deepak Chopra writes, "The most significant breakthrough is not contained in isolated findings but in a completely new worldview." Our current food worldview encourages us to look at food with binoculars. One moment we point them at protein, the next at carbohydrates, and then at fat — both in food and on our body. Viewed through such a restricted field of vision, we see food solely from a singular, biological perspective of "isolated findings."

But toss away the binoculars and instead view food through a kaleidoscope, and the multidimensional healing secrets of socializing, feelings, mindfulness, appreciation, connection, and optimal food emerge. And then, with the simple turn of the kaleidoscope, suddenly the healing secrets are distilled into the "four facets of food." In place of our interesting but limited binocular focus on food, stunning new nutrition insights are revealed; suddenly, subtleties that reflect physical, emotional, spiritual, and social nourishment are manifested. Viewed from such an interactive, ever-changing, multifaceted vantage point, food and nutrition become integrated, interconnected, and whole.

Rather than thinking about the four facets of food as a new diet or as more dietary dogma, as you read about them, I ask you to consider that they integrate our current nutrient-oriented view of food while also acknowledging the harder-to-measure healing dimensions of food, such as its link to emotions, spiritual well-being, and community. At their most meaningful level, the facets are independent of one another but also interdependent and profoundly interconnected. Once you begin to view food from this authentic, multifaceted framework, your entire relationship to food — and your perception about its power to heal holistically — will change at its core.

Facet One: Food for Physical Well-Being

If you've ever chosen a particular food after calculating its calorie content — with the intention of maintaining or losing weight — you've experienced the physical well-being facet of food. From this nutritional perspective, you're assessing food mostly as a "product" that is linked either to illness or to wellness. It tells us that what we eat is an amalgam of macro- (carbohydrates, protein, fat, fiber) and micronutrients (vitamins, minerals) that influence your health and well-being.

Viewing food from the perspective of physical health means analyzing it for its nutrient content, as animal or plant based, as processed, enriched (nutrients taken out have been added back), or fortified (new nutrients have been added to the food), as neutraceuticals (foods or components that provide medical or health benefits), as being irradiated (food has been exposed to radiation), or as a solution to be administered intravenously. This biomedical perspective includes studying the metabolism of food, what to eat, portion size, weight (of both food and your body), and the effect food has on the body (or on an ailment). Its aim is to use food and nutrition to treat, prevent, or reverse an ailment and to maintain bodily functions.

Facet Two: Food for Emotional Well-Being

Do you ever wonder why you crave carrot cake instead of a carrot when you're anxious? The facet of emotional well-being targets the effects your emotions and moods have on your food choices — and vice versa. Sometimes called "food-mood" research, nutritional neuroscience, or behavioral medicine, I describe the study of food and emotional well-being as psychological nutrition. This is because it is linked mostly to our emotions and food-related behaviors or disorders, such as food cravings, anorexia, bulimia, overeating, and subclinical eating disorders (SEDs), such as obsessions about food.

This emerging field of mind-body nutrition research assesses how food affects feelings via hormones (chemical messengers) that are released in the brain when we eat certain foods. The goal is to use food to achieve a desired emotional outcome and to understand how certain emotions and moods influence our food choices.

Facet Three: Food for Spiritual Well-Being

When you're not paying attention, are not fully conscious, food becomes merely something to eat. But if you blend the produce on your plate with "non-sense" — that which the ordinary senses cannot perceive — you're no longer eating only *for* your heart but also *from* the heart. When you eat with such conscious connection, regard, and appreciation, food becomes a path to spiritual well-being.

The core concepts of this spiritual food facet are connection and interconnection with your food through awareness of the interrelationship among living entities: soil, water, air, sun, plants, animals, ourselves, and those involved in bringing the food to our table (such as the farmer, the grocer, and the cook). Such spiritual nutrition explores the consciousness (degree of mindfulness, regard and appreciation, loving awareness, sense of connection, and so on) that we bring to our food. This philosophy and mentality is at the core of the food-related wisdom espoused by world religions and cultural traditions for thousands of years.

The desired outcome of the spiritual food facet is to perceive food (both plant and animal based) as an "equal," in that it contains the mystery of life as do we human beings and to appreciate the alchemy, the interconnection, the "oneness" inherent in food and eating.

Facet Four: Food for Social Well-Being

Think of your favorite food experience. Was it sharing food with some friends, family members, and coworkers, or were you dining at a table for one? This facet is about the benefits that food can bring when you're dining in a socially supportive environment.

Such social nutrition asks that we bring an "other-oriented" awareness (consciousness) to our meals by regarding the relationship among food, ourselves, friends, family, and others (such as cooks, farmers, and grocers), and that we be aware of our dining environment. It includes being conscious of whether you are dining alone or with others; acknowledging the setting (walking down the street, sitting in our car, watching TV); as well as taking in the aesthetics, such as the presentation of the food and the atmosphere of the room.

New Nutrition Insights

Why do we need new nutrition truths? A broader way of perceiving food and its role in our life? To expose the healing secrets and four facets of food? Because of one devastating fact: with our incredible knowledge about what's in our food, food-related health problems are not only continuing, they're getting worse. More of us die of diseases linked to malnutrition, poor diet, and obesity —

such as heart disease, diabetes, and hypertension — than all other illnesses combined, including cancer and AIDS. More than 55 percent of Americans are overweight, and as many as 40 percent of women and 24 percent of men are trying to lose weight at any given time. One and a half million people in this country suffer heart attacks every year, at least 60 million of us have high blood pressure and elevated cholesterol levels, 15 million are diabetic, and more than 9 million of us suffer from full-blown eating disorders.

I can personally vouch for these escalating health problems. During the twenty years I've been presenting seminars about optimal eating, conducting research, teaching, and writing about nutrition and health, I've met many individuals who truly believe they're eating well. But on closer scrutiny, it turns out that most are struggling with food-related issues: the majority are weight watching; others are calorie counting; still others are figuring the fat grams in their food. And all the while their weight problems, heart disease, and high blood pressure worsen.

What's gone wrong? Why aren't the incredible advances we've made in nutritional science during the twentieth century giving us the quality of life for which we've been striving and hoping? Why do so many of us find it difficult to apply nutritional knowledge to lose weight (and keep it off) or to prevent and reverse disease — even in the face of debilitating illness, even the possibility of death?

In other words, if our current knowledge about nutrition and our particular food focus aren't bringing the health transformations and benefits many of us have hoped for, what, then, will work? The answer is an integrative, comprehensive, total approach to food, an optimal eating program that nourishes body, mind, soul, and social well-being. These are the total-health healing secrets of food that I am thrilled to be telling you about throughout this book.

Eating by Number

In 1987, my father died abruptly, at age seventy-seven, of a heart attack. Several years later, my mother also died of heart disease; her death was due to congestive heart failure.

I knew a lot about nutrition then. Having worked as the nutrition educator with pioneering physician Dean Ornish, M.D., on his first clinical trial for reversing heart disease and later as the director of nutrition in Europe on a similar research project, I also knew a lot about lifestyle (diet, exercise, stress management, and group support, for example) and health, yet I still could not seem to find the "right" or "best" way to help my parents. It was during this frustrating period that I began to wonder if there was perhaps more to nutrition and food sciences than just the biological and technological examination of nutrients.

This nutrient-based approach to food — which I call "eating by number" — is a world with which we're all too familiar. Indeed, it's how we've been advised to eat each day: five or more servings of fruits and vegetables; less than 30 percent of calories from fat (10 percent or less to reverse heart disease); 1,200 mg. of calcium for women over fifty; 2,300 calories for men (less if you don't move much; more is okay with strenuous physical activity); 60 mg. of vitamin C; at least 280 mg. of magnesium, and so on and so forth.

Along with eating by number, we have mixed a scientific stew of jargon that was unfamiliar to most of us only a decade ago into our dietary lexicon. For instance, words such as *antioxidants* (protective substances that keep cells healthy) and *phytochemicals* (natural "pharmacies" in plant-based foods) now spice our food talk. We've made other great strides in our nutritional knowledge: today we take for granted that folic acid (a B vitamin) will lower the odds of heart disease for some, that carbohydrate-based foods (such as bread) can encourage calmness, and that avoiding hard, saturated fat may reduce the risk of ailments ranging from heart disease to various kinds of cancer.

But as useful as this information is, reducing food merely to fuel for our body and analyzing it as dietary details to be digested — both physically and intellectually — isn't the answer to optimal dietary self-care. For if it were, then surely most of us would make the recommended changes, and in the process, improve our health status. But this is not happening. Why isn't what we're doing working? Why haven't our incredible advances in nutritional science translated into optimal eating and improved health? As I know, and many of you know instinctively, food isn't only about nutrients and numbers. And people — even nutrition professionals — aren't computers who can memorize the nutritional data on cantaloupes, curry, or carrot cake and then use this information to choose the "best" meal. Consider a survey by researchers from New York University. When they asked dietitians attending a meeting of the American Dietetic Association in October 1996 to estimate the calorie and fat content of five typical restaurant meals (as well as in a glass of milk), the dietitians underestimated calories by as much as 50 percent and fat by 35 to 60 percent.

What do these results tell us? To me, they say we have a big problem that everybody's pretending doesn't exist. What is that problem? It's that we don't need more numbers, we need more meaning, other ways of relating to food so that each time we eat we have an enjoyable experience that nourishes our entire being. Instead, we're lost in a maze of measurements that don't adequately address our underlying food-related needs, such as the profound pleasure of eating, food-linked feelings, or the delight we take in dining with others.

The Old View: The Seeds of the SAD

Sometimes you have to go backward before you can move forward. In my exploration of the dynamics that led to our own Standard American Diet (SAD) and to such nutritional disregard and ignorance about food, I discovered five cultural forces. Although these "shifts" influenced our culture more than a century ago, they still form the basis of the disconnected dietary dogma we take for granted today. Here's a closer look at these health-robbing dynamics.

1. *Science supplants spirituality.* We first broke with religious tradition between the fourteenth and sixteenth centuries, a time of great intellectual and artistic achievement (the Renaissance). It was during the ensuing Enlightenment, though, that major scientific strides paved the way for the

scientific revolution that was to change the way we view the world (and food) forever. In the 1620s, Francis Bacon formulated the scientific method. Seemingly overnight, in lieu of seeing the world as an integration of visible matter (such as food) and invisible dimensions (such as feelings and spirituality), we started to measure, describe, and predict all natural phenomena.

Later in the century, Sir Isaac Newton's discovery of mathematical formulas that could accurately predict the movement of the planets jump-started a momentous paradigm shift in our worldview. Not only the planets but also our bodies began to be viewed as something that worked "like a clock."

How is this history lesson relevant to the way you perceive food today? Every time you purchase, say, a package of cereal, the nutrition information on the label is a reflection of the Newtonian belief that everything can be measured and reduced to a number. The end result? The timeless, highly regarded meaning in our meals has become obsolete.

2. *Nutritional science is born.* The genesis of perceiving food as something that could be counted and measured started in France in the eighteenth century when chemist Antoine-Laurent Lavoisier defined the *calorie,* a measure of energy in food. Then in the 1840s, German scientist Justus von Leibig isolated proteins, fats, carbohydrates, and minerals in food. But these discoveries didn't change our thinking about food much — until the Industrial Revolution and the development of separated food.

3. *Refined, processed food predominates.* Though roller mills — large cylinders that could crush wheat kernels and separate the flour, germ, bran, and other components of the grain — were patented in the 1750s, it wasn't until porcelain mills were introduced in 1870 that inexpensive white flour — in lieu of whole-wheat flour — became popular food for the masses. By the early 1900s, this separated food (what we now call "refined" or "processed") and ensuing nutrient loss resulted

in diseases of malnutrition (such as beriberi and pellagra) throughout England and America and also countries such as Japan and China, where the population had turned from brown rice to milled white rice. We now knew what to do with the nutrients discovered in the mid-1840s: enrich white flour food products by adding back four of the twenty-five nutrients lost in processing. In this way, we could lower the odds of deficiency diseases.

4. *Science saturates the kitchen.* In the 1880s and 1890s, American chemist Wilbur Olin Atwater encouraged Americans to apply the principles of the new science of nutrition to their family meals. A modern man who was a product of the scientific revolution, he wrote magazine articles telling us that food is fuel and that the body should be treated like a machine. Atwater was also the first person to create food lists containing the nutritive value of foods, lists that were published by the United States Department of Agriculture in 1885. Ultimately, Atwater defined the country's nutritional standards. Taking his scientific suggestions to heart, home economists (called "domestic scientists") of the time admonished homemakers to use the "new science" to create family meals that would be a well-balanced conglomeration of calculated and computed calories and nutrients.

Today, when you buy a magazine or read an article about the latest/newest/best/better nutrient or diet — and then try to incorporate it into your (or your family's) meals, you're following a tradition that began a century ago. This food-as-medicine approach is unique to America. Most cultures throughout the world do not relate to food as a "product" to be analyzed each time it's eaten. Rather, they enjoy food as the social, ceremonial, sensual delight it is.

5. *Puritan and Victorian values predominate.* Have you ever eaten a favorite food then proclaimed it to be sinful, bad, or illegal? Many of us regard food as a biological necessity to be feared, counted, or condemned. Such qualities projected onto food have their genesis in our Puritan heritage. The Puritans were

a sixteenth- and seventeenth-century English Protestant group that advocated a strict moral code and who regarded luxury or pleasure as sinful.

Then during the health-reform movement that ensued in the early nineteenth century, Victorian reformers such as graham cracker guru Sylvester Graham (who linked gluttony with evil) and cold cereal founder John Harvey Kellogg preached against gluttony and advocated a "right" way of eating. Indeed, author Michelle Stacey, writing in *Consumed: Why Americans Love, Hate, and Fear Food*, describes Victorian values as one of the "seeds of self-denial" that transformed our relationship to food as the twentieth century loomed.

Real-Food Manifesto

I'm very concerned about where these cultural forces have led us. And so are many others. As I write this sentence, a food revolution is in progress. I'm speaking of the backlash in America, and to a greater extent in Europe, against the globalization of McDonald's and what one Frenchman calls "multinationals of foul food." Is tampering with nature and food acceptable? Not for many Europeans, who refuse to buy "Frankenfood," produce that has been manipulated by American technology. But there are other technological, less visible food trends about which many are also concerned: neutraceuticals, irradiation, and more recently, the field of transgenics (turning foods into "vaccines" that enhance immunity).

Isn't it sad that our compartmentalized approach to food and our Standard American Diet have so distorted our relationship to food? We have a convention in this country that whatever's edible is food. But this isn't true for everyone. When friends from Europe recently visited my husband, Larry, and me, they commented constantly — and with amazement — about what passes as food or beverage in this country: Jell-O; tasteless white bread; powdered iced tea; huge servings of synthetic soft drinks; plastic-flavored, processed sweets; "dead," overcooked, over-salted vegetables; a plethora of fried fast foods — I could go on and on. Not only did they find these "foods" unappetizing, if truth be told, my European friends were appalled by the proliferation of American food "products."

Many Americans, though, readily welcome fake, "foul" food into their bodies. Somehow, with all our nutri-babble, we have forgotten what the experience of eating food is really about. We have forgotten that in some mysterious, alchemical way, food becomes one with us, and we with it — both literally and metaphorically, and that both food and we have and give life.

Before continuing, I want to take this moment to declare what food, real food is — and has been for millennia — before we turned it into something to study and dissect. Here is my declaration:

Declaration of Real Food

1. Real food is fresh.
2. Real food is natural.
3. Real food is whole.
4. Real food is nourishing.
5. Real food is healthful.
6. Real food's original integrity is intact.

I wrote this Declaration of Real Food because what passes today as edible isn't necessarily real food. Much of the time it's not nourishing, it's not natural, it's not fresh or whole, it's not healthful, and often its initial components have been destroyed. "Fake" food has become so imbedded into our nutritional landscape that we consider it part of normal nourishment — but it isn't. Most people throughout the world don't eat the way we do, nor is the typical American fare what we ate as we evolved as human beings. And we are paying for this diet with the diminishment of our health and quality of life.

The Meaning in Meals

In this book, I'll show you how to reap the health rewards of the healing secrets of food by relearning what real, optimal food is and how the social milieu, feelings, mindfulness, appreciation, and connection you bring to food and eating can contribute to your well-being.

The idea to season each meal with the healing secrets of food sprang from my sojourn into both state-of-the-art science and into what Huston Smith calls the wisdom traditions, major world religions (such as Judaism, Christianity, Islam, Buddhism, and Hinduism) and cultural traditions (such as yogic nutrition, the Japanese Way of Tea, Chinese food folklore, Native American food beliefs, and African-American soul food) that serve as guidelines for how to live (in our case, how to eat). Our spiritual ancestors took these dynamic, healing secret ingredients for granted — not only with food but with all life. When stirred together, they make a new nutrition stew spiced with meaning, feeling, regard, care, compassion, connection, love, community, divinity — and ultimately, enhanced health.

As you will see throughout this book, most cultures and religions relate to food as more than just sustenance. For instance, Native Americans have a tradition of fasting to connect with the life energy inherent in vegetables, plants, animals, and all life forms; African-Americans celebrate life and friendship by creating soul food with love; Tibetan monks turn food into art to reflect upon the impermanence of all life; Jewish people honor the sanctity of the life in both animal- and plant-based food; and Catholics and Episcopalians honor the divine through the bread and wine of Holy Communion.

Intuitively, over the centuries various cultures and religions have turned to food for more than sustenance for the body. They knew what modern researchers are beginning to conjecture: that bringing a broader, meditative awareness to food has powerful effects; indeed, when consciously cultivated, this awareness becomes a vehicle for connection to Mother Nature, the Divine, the mystery of life — and to health and well-being. When we lost this mind/body/spirit connection to food (and other aspects of life), our relationship to food became imbalanced and incomplete. The result is that many of us have deep food-related difficulties, ranging from confusion, anxiety, and fear to obsession, eating disorders, and cravings. Still others struggle with diet-linked ailments such as heart disease, osteoporosis, certain cancers, and being overweight.

Alchemy in Action

Ultimately, balancing your relationship to food, using your incredible human intelligence to look at more than food's caloric and nutrient content, is what will enhance your physical, emotional, spiritual, and social well-being in the long run. Doing so calls for seeing connections between food and body, mind, soul, and social well-being and making integrative eating — which includes the spiritual quest — an essential part of dietary self-care.

This approach is not as far-fetched as it may seem, for perhaps no science is more alchemical than nutrition. Indeed, the human body transmutes food into life-giving energy — which is alchemy in action. So is food's potential to give back to us the attention, intention, and regard we put into it. Although many of us perceive alchemy as medieval hocus-pocus about turning lead into gold, this perception is skewed. For alchemy truly was a profound marriage of science and spirituality. Its actual aim was for the alchemist to transmute from a state of "leaden" earthly awareness to one of "golden" spiritual perfection. And its core philosophy is that an underlying and all-pervasive energy or consciousness connects everyone with everything, all with all, mind with body, and biology with psychology.

The Broader View: Integrative Nutrition

In the 1970s, Harvard physician Herbert Benson, M.D., changed our view of mind/body medicine forever. With the publication of his book *The Relaxation Response,* he introduced the idea that meditation was good for our health. Up until that time, we believed that only Eastern mystics used this powerful healing technique for spiritual pursuits. Today, ideas about the healing benefits of meditation have become mainstream. Likewise, when former *Saturday Review* editor

Norman Cousins cured himself of chronic, progressive ankylosing spondylitis with laughter and large doses of vitamin C, we thought it impossible. Since then, scores of people have discovered his message: humor heals.

In *The Healing Secrets of Food* I aim to send a message similar to Benson's and Cousins's. It is a revisioning of nutritional health, a genuine alternative to the medical assumptions that still lie at the core of our modern approach to nutrition and health: that food is fuel and the body is a machine that needs the right mix of nutrients to be healthy. I impart this message by bringing ancient food wisdom into the twenty-first century and, conversely, by wedding modern science (delving into disciplines as diverse as nutritional anthropology, religion, psychology, quantum theory, biology, and social science) with ancient insights about food.

Larry Dossey, M.D., wrote in *Reinventing Medicine* that "we have stopped our investigation of healing well short of its potential." In the same way, we have limited our investigation of food and nutrition to a singular scientific framework, a reductionist perspective that reduces food to functional fuel and nutrients for our body. The healing secrets of food that you'll discover in this book are the foundation of a broader view, an integrative approach to food that may, ultimately, empower the investigation of nutritional science to live up to its potential.

Accomplishing this goal calls for nothing short of reclaiming the integrative nutrition heritage that has served humankind for millennia. What is integrative nutrition? It is a holistic approach to food and nutrition. Specifically, it is about the power of food to heal — not only physically but also emotionally, spiritually, and socially. Also, it is based on three worldviews about food and diet: Western nutritional science, Eastern healing systems that include nutrition (such as traditional Chinese medicine, Ayurveda, and Tibetan medicine), and timeless lifestyle wisdom about food (gleaned from world religions, yogic nutrition, the Mediterranean diet, and so on). Ultimately, integrative nutrition is not only about what to eat but also about how to eat for optimal health.

The aim of this book is to reexamine and redefine the healing powers of food within this integrative framework and to inform the world that we need not only to discuss the healing secrets but also to practice them daily. For when we do, we have the potential to heal our body, our emotions, our sense of spiritual connection, our social link to one another and communities, and potentially, our world and planet.

How This Book Is Organized

The process of integrative eating discussed throughout this book is both a personal journey and a health-enhancing adventure. In chapter 1, I introduce you to the six healing secrets of food. Chapters 2 through 7 are devoted to guiding you step-by-step through each of the healing secrets. The practical tips and personal stories in the "recipe" sections at the end of each chapter will give you the tools you need to flavor your meals with the healing secrets each time you eat. The more you practice them, the more you will open yourself up to the world within food and within yourself, helping you to find meaning — and optimal health — in each meal.

Chapter 8, "The Meal Meditation," will empower you to integrate and implement all the secrets. And the postscript celebrates their wisdom and awakens in us the ability to trust and listen to our hearts. Finally, to give you perspective on how well you are integrating the healing secrets of food into your everyday lives, I have included in the appendix "Your Integrative Eating Profile." And the bibliography provides more resources for the seeker in us all.

As you read each page, you'll come away with entirely new insights about food and nutrition. Beginning with your next meal, you'll know what it means to eat optimally — and you'll be awakened to the power of food to nurture your physical, emotional, spiritual, and social well-being.

chapter one

Out of the Dark Ages

The truth shall set you free, the Bible tells us. Each time you implement the nutritional truths in this book, you'll be set free from the tyranny of dieting, obsessing about food, and worrying about the best way to eat. When you familiarize yourself with the healing secrets of food spelled out in this chapter, confusion will turn to clarity.

Although your interest in food and nutrition may be to "eat well," to reduce the risk of illness, or to pursue the "perfect" diet or body, for many, food has become something that creates both physical and emotional havoc. We go on diets, overanalyze and obsess about food, turn to it as an enemy or friend, eat too much, eat too little, worry about it, avoid it, crave it, revere it, or believe that a particular nutrient will magically halt heart disease or cure cancer.

Yet even with such conscientious attention to food, we've become the fattest people in the world (along with the Pacific Islanders). I am disheartened and dismayed that in the face of this daunting statistic, we continue to pursue the "magic diet," the miracle supplement, the special, secret elixir that will keep us thin and heal us — effortlessly.

Our Magical Mystery Tour

The unrealistic, unrewarding, and frustrating way in which many of us relate to food can be illuminated by one of my favorite movies, *The Wizard of Oz*, and its many meaningful messages. When we think of this classic, beloved fantasy film, we remember Dorothy's attempt to return home "to her own backyard" and the companions she meets along the way: the indecisive scarecrow who needs "smarts," the cognitive tin man who hopes for a heart, and the meek lion who seeks courage. Much of the story is about the challenges they meet as they make their way to the Emerald City, believing the wizard will magically solve their physical and emotional problems.

In our ongoing quest for magical results from fad diets and our willingness to believe claims about substances (such as diet products) that are often aggrandized beyond what they are capable of delivering, are we not like Dorothy and her friends who sought to correct their limitations by seeking help from an illusory savior? "If you were really great and powerful, you would keep your promises," Dorothy admonished the Wizard when he reneges on his promise to grant their wishes. Isn't Dorothy's frustration similar to our own when yet another diet, another pill, another potion doesn't deliver the promised results? Doesn't Dorothy's sense of hopelessness about finding someone to solve her problems remind us of our own hopelessness about finding the magic mix of nutrients or the perfect diet to heal us?

The lessons in *The Wizard of Oz* suggest that the solution to our search for the optimal way to eat lies within us and our rich dietary heritage, that dietary wisdom and the best eating style have always been in our own backyards, in the depths of our own cultural, spiritual, and scientific traditions. In other words, food itself holds the answers for which we've been searching, but we've been looking in every direction except food and its timeless wisdom. Instead, some of us have turned to diet books, while others have been looking for answers by going to retreats and spas; still others have been pursuing practices such as meditation.

Regardless of our efforts, though, our trips to these various "wizards" aren't working as well as we'd like in helping us tap into food's healing powers. This is because we're trying to heal our body, mind, soul, and connection to community piecemeal. All the while, we're ignoring the solution in our own backyard: all six pieces of the healing secrets of food puzzle discussed throughout this book.

Creating Conscious Connection

Because our food-related health problems are both ongoing and worsening, it's a shame that we continue to walk down the same well-trodden food path. What we fail to realize is that many of society's problems stem from the fact that we are either physically isolated (watching TV, working alone at the computer, dining alone) or emotionally disconnected from one another, from the Divine, from the earth — and often from ourselves.

This physical isolation and emotional disconnection is also evident in our relationship to food. In our hurry-worry society, we no longer enjoy meals at the table, in quiet settings, with people we love, with food that's truly nourishing. After all, don't many of us eat while driving home, while standing at the kitchen counter, while strolling in a shopping mall, quickly, mindlessly? Aren't many of us focusing solely on flavor or nutrient content or constantly dieting? In this way, we're neglecting our spirit, we are destroying our souls.

Ultimately, our busyness and focusing solely on externals such as weight keep us from seeing a simple yet profound truth: we must connect with what we're eating, become one with its nourishing life force, or we may not survive. Consider this poem about the spiritual consequences of separation and disconnection from the primordial source of life, written by Sufi mystic and poet Jelaluddin Rumi in the thirteenth century:

Listen to the story told by the reed
of being separated.
Since I was cut from the reed bed
I have made
this crying sound. Anyone
separated from someone he loves
understands what I say:
Anyone pulled
from a source
longs to go back

(*The Illuminated Rumi,* translated by Coleman Barks)

It's a tragedy that we've become separated from the eternal source, the realm of ever-present love, the same primordial source from which both we and food evolved. The good news is that because the healing secrets of food have been with us for ages, we can relearn them and turn to them to reconnect with what is meaningful about food (and all aspects of life). After all, isn't this sense of connection to, and interconnection with, food at the core of what we're searching for when we window-shop for the best way to eat or pursue such popular spiritual paths as yoga and meditation? Aren't many who participate in the New Age movement trying to return to a place that people before us went to each time they ate? We, too, can visit this same spiritual abode by practicing the healing secrets whenever we're shopping for, cooking, or eating food.

Gleaned from insights derived from our evolutionary and spiritual ancestors, much of my integrative eating approach evolved from lasting, basic beliefs about food that have inspired and sustained humankind for centuries. Without thinking about it, our ancestors turned each "food moment" into a meaningful experience, a time to create conscious connection to the mystery of life inherent in both food and in us. Once you visit this wise, multifaceted culinary world, you may never want to return to today's limited view of food. As a matter of fact, you'll find that it's much easier to relearn the ancient food wisdom inherent in the healing secrets and to flavor your meals with these timeless values than to continue on the path of confusion and escalating isolation and illness.

The Six Healing Secrets

Because our current approach to nutrition isn't working well for so many of us, as a nutrition researcher, educator, and health journalist, it appalls me that so much of the literature in my field continues to focus exclusively on only one of the six secrets: what to eat. If the dice in Las Vegas casinos were fixed so that only the same side kept showing up every time you rolled them, everyone would scream "cheat!"

We are being cheated nutritionally. Food constitutes a six-part gift, but all we're hearing about is one thing. But this skewed perspective, focusing solely on the physiological aspects of food, has become the norm. I call our one-sided, limited view the Dark Ages of nutrition. We think that nutritional science is at its pinnacle, but in fact, most of us are still in the dark about what can most benefit us about food. This is because we're ignoring the most important elements of food and nutrition — the healing secrets of food — that have served humankind for centuries. They are:

1. Unite with others through food.
2. Be aware of your feelings before, during, and after eating.
3. Bring moment-to-moment nonjudgmental awareness to each aspect of the meal.
4. Appreciate food and its origins — from the heart.
5. Create union with the Divine by "flavoring" food with love.
6. Eat fresh, whole foods in their natural state as often as possible.

All these elements count — not just one or two in isolation. With this book, I hope to expose the injustice and partisanship of this one-sided view by insisting that the other sides of the "nutritional dice" get fair play. I'll show you how to eat optimally by revealing all sides of the dice — the healing secrets of food — the "nutrients" missing from the food charts.

From Secret to Celebration

As powerful as the healing secrets of food are, I am disappointed that experts — from food writers to dietitians and religious leaders

— don't learn, practice, and teach what these secrets have to offer, emphasizing their valuable health-giving properties and benefits every opportunity they get. I am disappointed that we consider only what can be measured in food, while we've forgotten that what is not so easily measured might be much more valuable to our health. I am disappointed that society as a whole isn't paying more attention to the healing secrets of food. Instead we choose to ignore a powerful truth: food has the ability to heal us in many ways — if we take the time to tap into its powerful healing properties.

I'm concerned that the healing secrets of food will remain secrets as long as we continue to insist that food is a two-dimensional issue: satisfying taste buds, or meeting nutritional requirements. Instead of yet another article about "fifty things you can do with Jell-O," we need to celebrate the secrets. Women's magazines, health magazines, and food and beauty magazines should all be touting the secrets, putting them on their covers, broadcasting them. Instead, food editors would have you believe that only pleasing your palate matters; many religious leaders would have you think that your relationship with God doesn't count when you eat, that it's present only when you're in formal prayer or devotion; and nutrition and food experts would have you focus exclusively on calories and nutrients. We're not seeing food's connection to others; its connection to our feelings; its connection to nature; its connection to God; and of course, its profound, multidimensional connection to ourselves. The end result is that food isn't satisfying, because our relationship to it is incomplete and disconnected from the whole of life.

Where, I wonder, is the meaning, the invisible satisfaction in our food? The human connection? The pleasure? The delight? The soul satisfaction? Where are the missing "secret ingredients," what philosopher Huston Smith calls "forgotten truth" about food and its meaning in our lives? Author Ken Wilbur articulates this dilemma of objective scientific truth versus underlying meaning that cannot be measured objectively. In his book *The Marriage of Sense and Soul*, he writes, "Science is clearly one of the most profound methods that humans have yet devised for discovering *truth*, while religion remains the single greatest force for generating *meaning*."

Our ancient ancestors understood instinctively the significance of putting meaning into meals. Throughout the centuries, people of many religions and cultural traditions have infused food with meaning in ways that are still evident today. For instance, devout Christians begin meals with a prayer of thanks; Indians refer to *bhoga,* a collective term for any food ingredient being used as an offering to God; with compassion for food animals as a guideline, Jewish dietary laws specify prohibited and acceptable food; and a reverence for, and connection to, nature and food is an integral part of Native American Indian beliefs.

When the meaning in our meals is lost, what's left is a list of rules and regulations that are not meaningful and therefore not motivating or sustainable. This truth became evident as my mom and dad struggled to overcome their heart problems. I knew they understood the heart-healthy dietary information I'd given them, but in retrospect, I realize that the underlying message was, "You *should* be eating differently. You *should* stop eating familiar and comfortable foods. You *should* assess and analyze what you're eating." Should. Surely what we should do or eat isn't a great motivator (nor is it emotionally appetizing). Indeed, the dictionary states that the word *should* implies obligation. Is this what food is really about? Is it something we're obligated to eat, to analyze, to weigh, to judge, to avoid, to crave, to overconsume, to underconsume, to control, to love, to hate, to fear, or to revere?

When we assess the vast nutritional resources of our culinary heritage and merge this wisdom with what modern nutritional science has to tell us, our relationship to food becomes integrative and therefore optimal. In lieu of being tossed around in a storm of nutrients and numbers, you become empowered to actualize an eating style that holds the potential not only to nourish your physical health but also to enhance your emotional, spiritual, and social well-being. Food becomes a celebration of life.

The Main Course

With this book, I'm calling for a renaissance — a reflowering of the way we view food and nutrition. This new view asks that we pay

attention to all the healing secrets — and to demystifying, understanding, and practicing them every day. I'm especially thrilled to
tell you about these long-lost healing secrets — not only because of
their timeless wisdom, but because they contain the answers we've
been looking for — but in all the wrong places.

Ultimately, their message is simple: the healing gifts of food are
available to us each time we eat. As a matter of fact, every time you
shop for, prepare, and eat food you have the opportunity to connect
with the life-giving, life-containing mystery inherent in food. These
activities are also opportunities to connect with loved ones, with the
earth, with life itself. In this way, you can heal not only yourself but,
ultimately, the planet.

PART TWO

The Healing Secrets of Food

chapter two

The Healing Secret of Socializing

Unite with others through food.

But now when I think of the...meals: the Sunday dinners in the formal salle à manger... the enormous suppers...when soufflés sighed voluptuously... and cold meats and salads and chilled fruits in wine and cream waited for us... no, when I think of all that, it is the people I see. My mind is filled with wonderment at them as they were then.

— M. F. K. Fisher, Long Ago in France

Sitting together around a table for meals is far more than a practical necessity. In its sacral character the sharing of food and drink is probably the most ancient ritual of mankind.

— *Manuela Dunn Mascetti and Arunima Borthwick,*
Food for the Spirit

I am excited to be sharing the healing secret of socializing, because not only does it show you how to turn dining with others into a balm for body, heart, and soul but it also reveals that meals can contain invaluable memories that help to heal what writer Elizabeth Cady Stanton describes as "the solitude of self." As you will see, when you unite with others through food — and your eating style shifts from a "me" mentality to a "we" awareness — you'll feel connected to something larger than your personal concerns, food related and otherwise. And when you do, you'll ignite the healing light of social connection.

As extraordinarily simple as the healing secret of socializing appears, beware: it is a two-edged sword in that can be both easy and difficult to implement. As many of you know, the demands of home, family, and career — and contending with cellular phones, pagers, and ongoing E-mail that keep us on call seemingly twenty-four hours a day — make it challenging to carve out some quality quiet time, let alone time to dine with others. Yet, once you learn — as I did — the amazing healing possibilities of this social nutrition secret, your body, mind, and soul will instantly begin to reap the benefits.

As you read this chapter, keep in mind that I qualify this healing secret with the suggestion that you unite with others through food *whenever it is feasible and possible.* My intent is not to give you more dietary dogma to follow rigidly. Rather, this book is designed to empower you to eat optimally as often as possible. Accomplishing this calls for keeping your food issues and health concerns in mind as this and all the other chapters reveal the multidimensional ways in which with whom, how, and what you eat influence your health. At the end of this chapter, I'll show you easy ways to bring this healing secret into your life each day, but for now, it's important for you to grasp the simple concept that dining in a socially supportive environment makes a difference to your health and well-being.

Dashboard Dining

What does it mean to unite with others through food? Simply put, it means putting interaction with others back into your dining experience. In this regard, the healing secret of socializing begins with being aware that our current food perspective is imbalanced and incomplete. The sole function of food isn't to provide fuel or the body to work, and eating isn't yet another mindless, functional, must-do chore to do "right." Rather, eating can be a health-enhancing, empowering, unifying, creative adventure when you share not only food but also camaraderie as you dine.

This approach is quite a contrast to the often isolated meals many of us eat while task stacking: doing other activities while eating. This includes driving alone in our cars, walking in a mall or down the street, working by ourselves in front of the computer, watching TV, or perhaps flipping through a magazine. Still others sneak snacks, glad that no one is around to witness the splurge.

As a matter of fact, we've gone from eating on the run to what futurist Tom Peters describes as taking our "food on the fly." Indeed, our task-stacking lifestyle has spurred the evolution of "dashboard dining," a phenomenon that's on the rise. With Americans currently eating about 20 percent of meals inside their cars — often between errands or meetings — the fast-food outlet, In-N-Out Burger, developed paper "laptops" so that you can keep your professional clothes clean while you're rushing a meal in your car on the way to work. Ever willing to meet Americans' growing dashboard dining needs, other businesses have joined the trend. For instance, automakers such as Saab have developed models with refrigerated glove boxes; Honda provides a pop-up table in the console. This eating-alone trend is escalating: with Burger King's Net-ready terminals, you can "log on and pig out" at your computer, writes James Daly, editor in chief of *Business 2.0*.

Our meals weren't always eaten on the fly. Before turning eating into an isolated experience replete with drive-through windows and fitting in food between an array of other activities, for tens of thousands of years, our ancestors most often ate in clans, bands, or tribes, with an intuitive understanding that their survival depended on eating this way. And when we were babies, given mother's milk or being bottle-fed, we took our nourishment while being held, in relationship with another person.

When I searched through the texts of the ancient wisdom traditions to explore how we ate before becoming so socially disconnected from both others and our food (see introduction), I learned that for every religion (such as Judaism, Christianity, Islam, Hinduism, and Buddhism) and cultural tradition (including yogic nutrition, African-American soul food, the Japanese Way of Tea, Chinese food folklore, or Native American food beliefs), food and eating have been intimately interwoven with our relationships with other people. Indeed, connecting with others through food is our social legacy, a refuge where memories reside, a nourishing world wherein traditions endure.

Most of us, though, not only do not pay much attention to how or with whom we're eating, but we also don't even believe that these two factors have anything to do with our health or well-being. But they do — and I am glad to let you know that both scientific research and the ideas contained in this book are shedding light on the healing power inherent in supportive social connection while dining.

The French Paradox

I vividly remember the moment when I realized that uniting with others through food was a potentially potent healing secret. It was when the enigma of the "French paradox" surfaced in the early 1990s. If you recall, research revealed that although aerobic exercise is unknown in France and smoking is a national pastime — as is a flood of relatively high-cholesterol, high-fat foods (such as cheese and butter-filled croissants) — the French seemed to have exceptionally low rates of heart attack. Not only is their heart attack rate 40 percent lower than that of fat-phobic Americans, but they outlive us by about two and a half years.

Stunned by the seeming contradiction of a high-fat diet and low heart attack rates, researchers around the world set out to solve this seemingly mysterious riddle. Over the years, many theories have surfaced. For instance, because the French often consume moderate amounts of red wine with meals, some attributed the metabolic mystery to the naturally occurring cholesterol-lowering resveratrol in wine. Others considered that there wasn't a French paradox after all, because of the way in which the French code their mortality data. More recently, the secret was attributed to the variety of French food itself — which includes lots of heart-healthy fruits and vegetables, minimal red meat consumption, olive oil in lieu of lard, less snacking, and other healthful key ingredients such as fish, onion, and garlic.

But while the French paradox may be partially explained by wine and diet, other researchers claimed it was due to a lifestyle that included ongoing social support: emotional, intellectual, and sometimes practical (assistance when needed) interaction with others — especially while dining. According to R. Curtis Ellison, M.D., chief of preventive medicine and professor at Boston University School of Medicine, the French "take longer to eat meals." Not only that, their long, leisurely meals are often enjoyed each day with three generations of family members as well as with friends. This provokes the questions: What are we Americans missing? Might dining in a pleasant, socially supportive atmosphere hold the power to heal?

The Significance of Social Support

Most of us know that eating in positive social surroundings is at the very least pleasurable. Yet the healing power inherent in a loving social atmosphere while dining continues to be an overlooked secret. One of the first and most intriguing studies to demonstrate the link between a socially supportive dining environment and health and well-being was published in the June 16, 1951, issue of the prestigious *Lancet*. An unusual experiment was conducted by a British nutritionist named Elsie M. Widdowson, who had the wherewithal to observe and record an extraordinary situation that developed in 1948 at two German orphanages shortly after World War II ended. Needless to say, this was a time of extreme trauma for the many German children who had been orphaned, a time when their sense of deprivation was exacerbated by food shortages and rationing.

When Widdowson arrived at the orphanages, she decided to take a year to study the effects of additional servings of food on the children's weight and height gain. During the first six months, the children at both orphanages received the exact same amount of rations; during the second six months, though, Widdowson gave children at one of the orphanages increased rations of bread, jam, and orange juice. Throughout the study — over a period of twelve months — she weighed and measured the height of the children every ten days. When the time came to look at the height and weight charts, Widdowson was puzzled. During the first six months — when all the children received equal food portions — children at one orphanage had gained significantly more height and weight than children at the other orphanage. The second six-month findings were equally confusing: those who had been fed more food gained less weight and height than those fed fewer food rations.

Widdowson pondered: Why had some children thrived while others hadn't — regardless of the amount of food they ate? When she observed the children's caretaker, she got her answer. Each group of children who had failed to gain weight and grow had been cared for by a strict disciplinarian who chose mealtime to administer public rebukes and to ridicule certain children. "By the time she had finished, the soup would be cold," writes Widdowson. "All the children would be in a state of considerable agitation, and several of them might be in tears."

The results of this study are amazing, because they suggest not only that the social atmosphere in which you eat can influence your health but also that dining with people who genuinely like you — and whom you like — can help you thrive even under adverse conditions. The key message: refrain from using the dinner table as a place to argue or to scold if you want to improve your physical and emotional well-being.

The Magic of the Midnight Meal

One morning while reading an article in a local newspaper, I got another clue about the emotional ways in which social satisfaction while dining can heal. While skimming the paper, I found myself riveted by an article titled "Midnight Supper: Spontaneous Party at the Witching Hour." Written by Lois Maclean, a then-unemployed, forty-something woman, "Midnight Supper" is a story about something very unusual that happened to her and her husband at 10:30 on a depressing Tuesday night. As they were considering whether to go "into a full-tilt harangue about everything that was wrong with [their] life," they received a phone call from Bradley, an old friend who had recently wed a woman from Hong Kong named Suk Wah; Brad was calling to invite them over for a midnight supper at a villa where he and Suk Wah were house-sitting.

Although Maclean and her husband were "awed by the very concept," taking their friend up on the invitation meant a half-hour drive at 11:00 on a weekday night across the long Richmond Bridge. They went anyway. As Maclean described it: "We threw on our jackets and hit the freeway, already feeling more interested in life." When they entered the villa, Maclean described the instantaneous hospitality and meal that manifested: "Bradley and Suk Wah handed us shrimp chips and flutes of champagne from their wedding.... At a cluttered table in the bright kitchen, we dispatched a giant bowl of Suk Wah's Chinese spaghetti, fragrant with ginger and dried shiitake mushrooms. Afterward, we curled up with cups of herb tea." Explained Suk Wah as she handed around the teacups: "midnight supper is a Chinese custom. We celebrate the magic of the night."

What impact did this satisfying social connection have on Maclean's mood and mental state? She and her husband "went home at around two in the morning, sated with simple food and simple kindness, our malaise dispelled. When we awoke in the morning, we felt...tired but satisfied, refreshed and a lot lighter of heart."

It is one thing to eat; it is another to dine on lovingly prepared food with good friends. For when we do, not only is our appetite nourished, but somehow our soul too is satisfied and we become "lighter of heart." When I had the pleasure of talking with Suk Wah Bernstein, I learned that her idea to "celebrate the magic of the night" with friends evolved from New Year rituals she had celebrated with her family during her childhood in Hong Kong. "China's ancient folk religion has a god for just about everything," she told me, "and on the eve of the Chinese New Year, all of them come to inspect us." By preparing a special midnight meal, the family welcomes both these hundreds of gods and the new year by gathering around and sharing an elaborate midnight meal; it is a truly festive family occasion.

Communing with Food

Wisdomkeepers is both the name of a book and a term used by authors Steve Wall and Harvey Arden to describe Native American spiritual elders, "the Old Ones." Over the centuries, wisdom keepers from cultures worldwide have intuited and encouraged the healing potential that may be ingested when we dine in an enjoyable social atmosphere. Consider Native Americans' social link to food. It was so all-encompassing that along with the earth and sun and most other aspects of nature, they perceived food itself as an actual family member. This is evident by the way in which the Senecas refer to their staple foods of corn, beans, and squash as the "Three Sisters," their "Supporters."

Uniting with others through food is also integral to Christianity. Indeed, the Last Supper — a Passover meal — shared by Jesus and his disciples became the most momentous meal in the history of Christianity, perhaps the world. As Christianity evolved, the sharing of the bread and wine of the Eucharist (transforming — either literally or symbolically — Jesus' body and blood into bread and wine) was related to a regular meal that early Christians would share together at an "open table" in their homes in communion with other faithful believers, regardless of their sociological or economic background. In "house churches," these early Christians ate, essentially, a potluck meal; then they observed the Eucharist together.

When Jesus was alive, sharing food had more significance than it does now. Sitting down and sharing a meal with someone signified that you accepted that person as an equal. Such a symbolic act, for instance, was manifested when Jesus dined not only with his disciples but also with tax collectors and sinners. Even after his resurrection, Jesus eats with his disciples, again signifying equality, an open table that doesn't discriminate. Today this tradition continues as Catholics take the Eucharist in communion with others.

If our past contains a single culinary theme, it's uniting with others through food. Perhaps nowhere is this more evident than in Judaism's teachings, which are resplendent with centuries-old, universally accepted concepts about food designed to make our meals heartwarming social occasions. For instance, for more than thirty centuries, devout Jews have taken great pleasure in sharing food — not only among themselves to honor and to connect with their past but also with others who are hungry. "In this way," writes author Claudia Roden in *The Book of Jewish Food,* "[social unity] is one of the great bonds of Jewish and community life."

Consider the Jewish Sabbath, a holy twenty-four-hour period that's been celebrated by Jews since biblical times. During this special time — which begins on Friday exactly eighteen minutes before sunset and ends on Saturday evening after dark — work and everyday activities are prohibited. Instead, devout Jewish families make it a point to stop the hustle and bustle of the week and instead partake of the Sabbath meal with family members and friends.

The concept of social connection through food is so all-encompassing that many Muslims actually define Islam as a social religion, with food playing a big part in bringing others together under its social auspices. Believing that the blessing received isn't only the food but also the company, Muslims espouse both eating with others and sharing food with others. The underlying intention was that the aroma of food while it cooked should encourage neighbors to come by and share the meal. In this way, framed in a feeling of kinship, Muslims may be brought together in the name of Allah (the Supreme Being in Islam) and together enjoy the meal in a devotional, loving context.

Reconsidering Rabbit Food

With uncanny foresight, wisdom keepers throughout the ages seemed to have anticipated the health benefits of social nutrition that were to be revealed by scientific discoveries made centuries later. For instance, one groundbreaking study, conducted by Dr. R. M. Nerem at the University of Texas, suggests that rabbits who ate while being cared for and regarded (what I describe as "eating from the heart") experienced some sort of mysterious alchemical change in the way in which they metabolized potentially artery-clogging food.

Here's what happened. To learn about the effect diet has on the development of coronary artery disease (CAD), researchers fed rabbits high-cholesterol, artery-clogging rabbit chow. But when it came time to tally the results, they found that some rabbits' arteries weren't clogged with plaque — even though they'd all been fed the same high-cholesterol foods. In fact, this healthier group displayed 60 percent less plaque. Unable to explain why some rabbits showed less evidence of the beginning stages of heart disease than others, the researchers decided to trace each step of the study.

Upon inquiry, they found that the rabbits in the cages stacked in the middle fared better than those in the higher or lower cages. When they asked the research assistant about this, she said that when she fed the rabbits, she had taken out the rabbits in the middle cages so she could pet, cuddle, and talk to them each day as she fed them. Apparently, it was harder for her to reach the rabbits that had been placed in the lower or higher cages; as a result, these rabbits received normal laboratory animal care — minus being talked to and touched while fed. Finding it difficult to believe that contact from the caretaker could make such a difference in the condition of the rabbits' arteries, the researchers replicated the study in a much more controlled fashion. Again, the results were the same: the arteries of the rabbits who were talked to and touched while eating exhibited less coronary artery disease.

As with the orphanage study, such results imply that a loving, supportive presence (and consciousness) while eating not only might help us thrive, it may also inhibit disease. At its core, the message in our meals is that love matters, and that when love is present while we're eating, it mysteriously connects us to other living entities — whether they be orphaned children, animals, or food itself.

The Healing Web of Relationships

Does positive social connection while eating also serve as a buffer against illness for people — regardless of whether the food is healthful? Years before the rabbit study, researchers answered this question when they conducted a fascinating study with Italian Americans who lived in Roseto, Pennsylvania. The researchers chose Roseto because of the extraordinarily low rate of coronary heart disease among its population compared to that in similar surrounding communities.

Studied for more than fifty years, most Rosetans lived on traditionally high-fat, high-cholesterol Italian sauces, sausages, and other potentially artery-clogging, heart disease–linked fare. Given this, scientists were perplexed about why the rate of heart disease, and the mortality from heart attacks, remained low in Roseto in spite of this diet, especially when compared to the relatively high rate of heart disease in nearby towns.

As this long-term study progressed, the rate of heart disease began increasing in Roseto until it equaled that of the general American population. What had changed? Upon closer scrutiny, the researchers realized that when the study began, it wasn't uncommon to find three generations of Italians living under one roof; close family ties and community cohesion were the norm. But as the Italian American children moved away from Roseto, the community's cohesion began to decrease. Roseto's traditional close-knit family and community structures weakened. Along the way, the commitment to religion, relationships, and traditional values also lessened a way of life that had united Rosetans since they'd migrated to America in 1882. Again, research revealed that strong, nurturing social ties, when wrapped around the food we eat, may hold the power to preserve more than a way of life that has been espoused by wisdom keepers for thousands of years. The implications? Even if we eat potentially heart-harming food, strong social bonds may actually prevent illness by somehow changing the way in which we metabolize food. I am not, of course, espousing that it is "safe" to consume high-fat, unhealthful foods as long as you're eating them with people you like!

Such studies aren't the only ones to suggest that dining with others in a nurturing environment may enhance health. In recent years, the link between social support and health status has become a major focus of research. Although the following studies aren't specifically food–oriented, nonetheless they strongly suggest that the healing web of relationships is powerful medicine.

- In the 1980s, graduate student Erica Friedmann discovered that people who survived heart attacks tended to be pet owners. Since that time, other studies have confirmed that the unconditional affection that animals offer seems to help pet owners with a variety of ailments — from lowering blood pressure to increasing the odds of recovering from a heart attack.
- Dr. Berkman and his colleagues' Alameda County study, which followed seven thousand men and women in northern California, found that those with weak social and community support systems were more than three times more likely to die than their socially connected counterparts. This fact remained true in spite of unhealthful lifestyles. Interestingly, those who lived the longest had both strong social ties as well as a healthful lifestyle.
- In 1989, yet another landmark study, by David Spiegel, M.D., and colleagues at Stanford Medical School, revealed that women with metastatic breast cancer who participated in weekly support group sessions lived twice as long as women who didn't participate in support groups.

Psychologist and researcher Jeanne Achterberg, speaking at the Institute of Health and Healing at the California Pacific Medical Center in San Francisco, summarized the link between social support and health this way: "Lack of social relationships constitutes the major risk factor in health, one that is even greater than smoking. Persons who are considered to be in a light-filled social network...are at less risk for high blood pressure, elevated cholesterol, heart disease, tuberculosis, accidents, psychiatric disorders, complications with pregnancy, and on and on." In other words, a strong social support system, the healing web of relationships, appears to be a major predictor of health, longevity, and mortality.

Reclaiming Your Social Nutrition Heritage

Societies have passed down the importance of the union of food, love, and positive social interaction from generation to generation. My friend Michelle, who grew up in Mexico City and moved to the

United States at the age of eighteen, experienced firsthand during her formative years what it was like to dine with her loving, large family. During her childhood years in Mexico, she lived in a culture where dining with others was — and still is — a deeply held value and custom.

Consider a typical Sunday for Michelle when she was a child growing up in Mexico. The entire family — adults and children, cousins, parents, aunts, uncles, and grandparents — got together for the midday meal, which in Mexico is called dinner. Often hosted by the family matriarch — either the grandmother or mother — the gathering sometimes began around breakfast time. After breakfast, the women decided what they'd make for dinner, which usually included soup as a first course, salad as a second course, a main dish that often consisted of vegetables, rice, and meat, then perhaps a tray filled with fresh fruit for dessert.

While the women prepared the meal, some men played soccer in a nearby field; others might fix bicycles or toys; meanwhile, small children played inside the house. At about 3:00 P.M., the entire family — often fifteen or more people — sat around the table to eat, chat, laugh, and enjoy the meal. Afterward, as the women cleaned up, they reminisced about the "old days" while sharing stories of their youth. At about 6:00, the various family members departed for their respective homes.

Did anyone ever eat alone? Not often, perhaps only when a person arrived home late from work. Says Michelle: "I believe that my love and appreciation of sharing fresh homemade meals with others comes from growing up with this tradition. I liked yakking with the family over food, and catching up on each other's lives. Those weekly get-togethers always gave me a warm, cozy feeling. When you share a major meal with family each week, it's a way of keeping connected with people you love."

In *Celebrating the Impressionist Table,* author Pamela Todd describes just such a vanishing and vanished social life, captured forever in canvases filled with sunlit scenes of food-centered celebrations and friendships: "Today [these paintings] evoke in us a feeling of well-being and a tinge of nostalgia for a time when love and light and good companionship — often cemented at the table — were elevated above the petty commercial concerns of everyday living," writes Todd.

Yet as a contrast, in the United States today, it's becoming more and more common to eat alone, to relate to food as a necessary, functional part of life, something to fit into our busy schedules. This mentality has even infiltrated our language. How many times do we hear: "I'm just going to grab something on the way home," "Don't hold dinner; I have to work late," or "Sorry I have to eat and run." The end result: whichever way you turn the dining table, it's still devoid of people.

Not only is there no time like the present to do something about the loneliness that permeates our culture, there is no better opportunity to do something about it than each time you eat. To access the social salve of dining with others, when I give presentations, I often ask people to think about how they feel in their soul during those quiet, often lonely times while going home after work. How would they feel if they knew that their grandmother had been preparing dinner all afternoon; if they knew that when they arrived home, they'd sit down to eat with their children, spouse, and grandparents? Then, perhaps after they ate the freshly cooked food while catching up on each other's lives neighbors who lived nearby would drop by to chat and share some dessert. Smiles and pleasurable sighs at the prospect are the usual response.

Implementing the healing secret of socializing each time you eat is one way you can take positive, constructive action not only to heal your relationship with food but also to correct the culture's unbalanced perception of the role of food and to reclaim your heritage. By putting into action the social and other healing secrets of food discussed in this book, you're positioning yourself not only to digest food's healing social nutrients but also its emotional, spiritual, and physical benefits.

Setting the Social Table

For some, uniting with others through food may seem simple; others might perceive it as a unique challenge. In actuality, dining with people in a pleasant atmosphere is part of our unique heritage as human beings. Whether eating together as a member of a tribe or clan or more recently during birthdays or weddings, we've been turning to food to enjoy or celebrate with others for millennia. As a matter of fact, some experts believe that this tradition became less common only when central heating evolved, and families no longer needed to gather together in the kitchen to stay warm.

Bringing social nutrition back into your life is especially easy, because it calls for making some minor shifts in what you're already doing. What follows are some suggestions for integrating social ingredients into your daily meals and for making social dining a more intimate and integral part of your life each day.

❧ *Set a table for two.* If you're dining alone, "socialize" by placing a photograph of someone you love on the table. As you sit down to eat, conjure up favorite food memories you've shared: perhaps some exceptional pasta primavera served in a favorite restaurant, the time you savored a piece of choice chocolate together, or a special summer potato salad you all enjoyed at a family picnic. Or does the fresh fruit you're having for dessert remind you of the blueberries you picked together during a walk in the country?

Here's another option: if you have a pet — such as a cat or dog — feed your pet first so you can feel connected to it while you're eating.

❧ *Take a social nutrition break.* When my husband and I worked on a clinical research project at a medical university in Europe, we would often join our colleagues for lunch at the local cafeteria and socialize over a simple salad or soup. Every office lunch, snack, or coffee break is an opportunity for you to access the healing secret of socializing. Whether you're "brown-bagging" it with a tuna sandwich or dining on a simple mixed salad you purchased at the local deli, when you're at work, why not make it a point to have lunch with coworkers? Or, in the afternoon, take a social nutrition break by enjoying a cup of yogurt, freshly popped popcorn, or herbal tea with like-minded coworkers. Ultimately, eating with colleagues is an opportunity to build relationships instead of yet another activity that you do alone at the office.

❧ *Finesse family fare.* A recently widowed father who was raising two preteen boys by himself told he realized that his sons and he weren't really eating together. Rather, it was typical for them to eat take-out pizza while watching TV. To change this pattern, he began to prepare more homemade meals whenever possible (macaroni and cheese with a tall glass of tomato juice were favorites) and to turn off the TV while eating. Soon he began looking forward to sitting around the dining room table with his sons and sharing stories about the day.

In the same spirit, if you, your spouse, and your children have busy schedules, is it possible to commit to one or two mornings to having breakfast together? Perhaps you can prepare pancakes, while others can contribute by organizing the toppings, such as yogurt, raisins, and chopped walnuts. Fresh-pressed orange juice and a fantastic fruit salad are other quick and easy — but special and tasty — options.

❧ *Create a social Sabbath.* At a seminar I gave, a devout Jewish woman told me that my talk about social nutrition had struck a chord. About fifty years old and divorced with grown children away at college, she realized that she ate alone too often and that she deeply missed both preparing and sharing meals with loved ones — especially Friday night Sabbath meals. Her solution? She planned to begin having a weekly potluck meal at her home with some special friends on Friday night.

If you used to observe the Sabbath but "just don't have time anymore," try bringing it back into your life. Or in the spirit of the Sabbath, initiate your own Friday night potluck get-together with special friends or family. It doesn't have to be time-consuming to create a dish for a potluck meal. For me, when time is an issue, I might make some sweet potato soup — served warm in the winter or chilled in the summer. Or, if you have the time, consider making fruit pies, prepared with varieties of seasonal fruit: plums, apricots, and cherries in the spring; peaches and blueberries in the summer; apples and pears in early fall.

❧ *Consider "soulful" dining.* Because slaves were forbidden to talk with one another or to socialize while working in the fields, preparing and eating soul food provided a joyous opportunity to spend time together. In this way, meals became social occasions that offered comfort to heart, body, and soul. "Eating soul" can be social in yet another way: because it's recipeless (slaves weren't allowed to learn to read and write), learning to "cook soul" has become an art that has been handed down from generation to generation during time spent together in the kitchen.

Some basics brought from Africa are goobers (peanuts) and benne (sesame seed paste), while meager food rations on the plantations were stretched by foraging for edible wild greens, wild onions, and wild roots, such as potatoes. Today, soul food is still simple — and socially satisfying — fare. In this light, consider having a soul-food fest. Ask an elderly aunt for a favorite family recipe, then prepare it and invite her and other family members over to enjoy it. Or ask some friends to come over to share and prepare some simple soul food dishes that, of course, are recipeless. Some suggestions: spiced mustard greens, corn bread, and a mixed vegetable and bean stew.

❧ *Connect with community.* Ultimately, the healing secret of socializing is about connection with self, family, friends, neighbors, environment, and community — with food as the unifying flavor. Wouldn't it be exciting if communities started to have potluck dinners so that everyone wouldn't have to continue eating alone? On a weekly, monthly, or annual basis, community members could get together for potluck meals by meeting in homes, community centers, synagogues, or churches or by creating food-focused street festivals.

Or in the spirit of the Chinese New Year, during any day of the work week, the holiday season, or on New Year's Eve, what about inviting over some special friends to share conversation and a candlelit meal of *zai* (the Chinese character for vegetarian food)? For example, serve pasta with a simple salad, veggies over rice, and some seasonal, sliced fruit or a sweet, with tea.

Recipes for Socializing

Whether you use one, some, or all the above suggestions for uniting with others through food, you'll be setting in motion the potential to heal not only your own body and soul but also the social well-being and fabric of our whole society. Here are some insights into traditional social bills of fare that have served humankind for millennia — and some not so traditional social ones that I have created over time.

❧ *Hindu wedding feast.* I first became aware of the far-reaching social significance of the Hindu wedding feast one afternoon when I was browsing through a fairly old (perhaps published in the 1950s) Indian cookbook. As I flipped through the pages, I came across a recipe for four, then eight, then — completely unexpectedly — for eight hundred! When I read the text, I learned that it was common for a Hindu wedding feast in India to include enough food for the entire village — which could include a community of eight hundred — or more!

In the same spirit, when my friend Nutan (from Mumbai, formerly Bombay) married, she and her family created a gracious afternoon buffet — held in a Hindu temple — to be shared by perhaps 150 close family members and friends. The dozen or so dishes ranged from papadum (a lentil-based crisp thin bread) and pullao (a saffron-flavored rice dish) to cilantro chutneys and keer (a rich rice pudding). Believed to enhance digestion, lassi, a buttermilk-based beverage, is served afterward. Traditional wedding sweets in India do not include a wedding cake; rather, they are usually a blend of milk, sugar, fruit, or nuts.

But such a feast was only a warm-up for what was to come: an evening reception at a restaurant for more than a thousand people. With perhaps twenty different dishes, this evening buffet was yet another expression of blessings and joy to the couple and the invisible link of love that unites the couple with family, friends, favorite foods, and festive feelings.

❧ *A birthday "breakfast."* Cake may not be part of the Hindu wedding feast, but for Westerners, it's a must when it comes to sharing birthday wishes with friends and family. The tradition of birthday parties began centuries ago in Europe as a deterrent to evil spirits, believed to be attracted to people on their birthdays. To protect the person having the birthday, friends and family would drop by, bringing good thoughts and wishes. Giving gifts was thought to be an even more effective strategy to ward off the evil spirits.

Today, such concerns have disappeared. Instead, many of us welcome our birthdays with a sense of expectation and exhilaration, not unlike that of being a child on Christmas morning. At least for the day, our life is pregnant with possibilities: surprise presents and celebrations, a cascade of good wishes, and candles burning on our birthday cake.

To keep early-morning birthday exhilaration from losing its glow, Larry and I have created our own special birthday ritual over time; our birthdays are truly full of pampering and bliss. We always begin by opening presents. Then the ensuing all-day celebration may include being whisked off to a romantic bed and breakfast, a walk in nature, a kayaking adventure, a surprise party, a massage, spa treatments, or a theater event … and always … a gourmet dinner and a special birthday cake. On one of these mornings of blessed indulgence, as I was opening my presents, I heard a knock on the door; it was probably only around 7:00. When I opened the door, nobody was in sight, but when I looked down, my eyes lit on an almost surreal scene: a perfectly round — but not too large — dark chocolate (my favorite) birthday cake, set on a tray that held a white plate, white doily, white lace linens, and a white birthday card. What an exquisite work of art, I thought appreciatively, while at the same time realizing that this was the latest creation of my artist friend (and neighbor) Donna Wallace, who lived next door. Lighting some candles while singing "Happy Birthday," Larry and I took a moment to savor a sliver of the enticing chocolate treasure; in our hearts, we were dining with Donna too.

❧ *Brunch in "Paris."* At one time or another, most of us have had the impulse to escape our daily dining routine and seek out a social, ceremonial, and sensual food experience. Such a fantasy took hold of me one Saturday morning, but when I invited Larry to participate, the dream retreated for a moment when he told me he was on deadline for a grant he was writing. Still, the craving would not go away, so I decided to create my own spontaneous social milieu and meal. Given my mood, the only place that would bring the satisfaction I craved was Paris; the only acceptable food would be food prepared with the élan and sensibility of a French feast. This meant that I would tarry over the foods' tantalizing tastes, savor the scents that surfaced, then linger over the café au lait. The satisfaction, I knew, would come from the attention to detail, the appreciation of both atmosphere and ingredients, and the regard for the social fabric inherent in food and eating.

We live in a small coastal town in northern California, and although it was summer, the early-morning fog created a gray, cashmere-like mist that blanketed our water view. I felt comforted and cozy as I walked into our guest room. Perfect — in my imagination, I would turn it into a Parisian bed and breakfast. Still ensconced in the fog, I lit some candles, turned on two table lamps to the lowest light setting, set the portable heater on an intense but low and silent setting (my improvised version of a fireplace), took out an antique tray, puffed up the pillows, spread a soft cotton quilt over the bed, and placed a just-delivered crisp copy of the *New York Times* on top of the quilt.

My next chance to create my meal presented itself when I walked into the kitchen. While Larry worked away at the kitchen table, I surveyed my culinary options: it would be easy to make my own delectable, delightful version of the typical French breakfast of juice, a croissant or baguette, and café au lait. My menu would be a variation, though: a fresh fruit smoothie, my favorite bread and spread, and café au "soy" (I typically drink soy milk).

To begin, I poured some orange juice into a blender (perhaps one-third cup), then I added a potpourri of fresh, frozen pieces of various fruits, all of which we had previously purchased at our local farmers' market, cut up into bite-size pieces, bagged, and placed in our freezer. My fruit medley consisted of a sprinkling of grapes and pieces of pineapple, apricots, peaches, strawberries, and banana. After adding a teaspoon of vanilla for more flavor and then water to thin the fruit mixture, I buzzed the colorful mixture in the blender for about thirty seconds. Then I poured a serving of the frothy, light-pink smoothie into an elegant wine glass, reflecting that I would enjoy the rest throughout the day. Perfection.

To prepare the bread, I sliced a piece from a round, fresh loaf of whole wheat–walnut sourdough bread (a staple in our home). Then I placed it in the toaster oven and watched as the heating coil turned orange. When the bread was toasted, warm, and fragrant, I placed it on a plate, drizzled a thin layer of tahini (sesame butter) on it, then infused it further with flavor by adding a dollop of chunky ginger jam.

About this time, the water for the café au soy came to a boil. I poured the hot water into a French press, which already contained a tablespoon of freshly ground (I used our automatic coffee grinder) decaf French roast coffee. After it had brewed for several minutes, I filled half of a large cup (a special café au lait cup I had bought in Paris when I had taken Larry there for his birthday several years ago) with the coffee; then I filled the rest of the cup to the brim with my favorite, warmed-up soy milk.

The last step: I placed the smoothie, toast, and café au "soy" on the serving tray, which by now also held a white, crisply folded, cloth napkin (usually used for company only). It was an easy effort. In less than fifteen minutes, I was seated on the bed in my toasty, warm guest room (my French B and B), sipping the smoothie and café au soy, enjoying the richly flavored bread, and reading the paper. At the same time, I could hear Larry rustling papers in the nearby dining area, where he was working. At that instant, I felt total, food-linked social satisfaction. It was a feeling similar to the one I'd had when, searching for the perfect bistro in Paris around dusk, Larry and I had made the right turn into the right restaurant. Instantly after entering, we found ourselves in a bustling and gleaming eatery, resplendent with lively but low chatter and inhaling the mingling of scents from meals that had satisfied both souls and the senses for centuries.

Reflecting on this former — and my current — "perfect meal moment," I finished the smoothie, then took another bite of the fragrant, ginger-spiced bread. Cupping the café au soy cup in both hands to revel in its warmth, I took another sip of the bittersweet brew. By this time, the sun was blazing through the early morning fog, which was beginning to lift outside my window. In its place was the familiar "Shangri-la" view of mist, mountains, water, sky, and otherworldly lighting that I knew I would never take for granted. Absolutely, I thought, I've created the social milieu and meal I so desired.

Sipping my coffee, I reflected on the pleasure imparted by

enjoying favorite foods in the company of others — whether the union is literal, in memory, or based on a preferred mood and atmosphere. Feeling celebratory, I toasted all those who had made it possible for me to enjoy this meal as well as our ancestors and the culinary wisdom they've passed along over the centuries: "Thank you for inventing the soul-satisfying delight that comes alive each time we enjoy a meal with others." The pleasure is all-encompassing, no matter where, or with whom, I'm dining — either literally or in my imagination.

chapter three

The Healing Secret of Feelings

Be aware of feelings before, during, and after eating.

With all that we now know about the food/mind/mood connection...
you can begin to select [food] that will...modify your moods
and...make you a more effective, motivated, and perhaps
even more contented individual.

— *Judith Wurtman,* Managing Your Mind and Mood through Food

I am delighted to tell you about the healing secret of feelings, because it invites you to enter into a dance between the food you eat and the feelings you feel. The elements of this dynamic dance duo are an awareness of the effect your feelings have on your food choices and the influence your food choices have on your feelings.

Becoming accomplished in doing this dance calls for being aware of feelings before, during, and after eating. Learning the steps isn't always easy, but I've found that it's well worth the effort. Once you're familiar with this food-mood dance, you'll experience the incredible interconnection between what you eat and how you feel. Along the way, food and eating become guides for balancing your feelings, celebrating the majesty of your meals, even transforming your relationship to food.

Later in this chapter, I'll give you practical tips for using food and feelings to your advantage each time you eat, but right now, I'm suggesting that if you pause to sense how you feel before, during, and after eating, you can take control both of your emotions and of what and how much you eat. Viewed from this perspective, each food you choose to eat can become a chance to fine-tune your moods and emotional health. And as it does, what and how we eat become a path to self-understanding and a tool for nurturing our emotional well-being and ultimately for enhancing the quality of our life.

The Real Challenge

Accessing the potent power that food has on your feelings and overall emotional well-being isn't always easy. Teasing out the emotions that manifest after you eat requires a subtle refocusing of attention — a shift of mind and heart, a new way of communicating with both yourself and your food. The real challenge, though, is that activating and benefiting from your feelings before, during, and after eating calls for acknowledging and accepting that, ultimately, you need to be willing to be alone with yourself and your feelings.

An experience I had years ago led me to this insight. When I was a teenager, I began to smoke cigarettes. Then, sometime during my early twenties, I decided to quit. I didn't do it for health reasons, though. Rather, I quit because a boyfriend at the time realized that whenever I was anxious about something, I would light up. And I didn't want to be so transparent.

Tossing my last pack of cigarettes into a dumpster was the easy part. I even found it manageable to get through the first few days and weeks while overcoming my addiction to nicotine. However, during this time, I realized that whenever I spoke with someone (sans cigarette), I not only had to figure out what to do with my hands now that I was no longer keeping them busy with a cigarette but I also needed to readjust where I focused my eyes. Now that I could no longer divert my eyes by searching for a cigarette, matches, or an ashtray — or by mindlessly daydreaming into the cigarette smoke — I actually had to relearn how to have a conversation while sustaining eye contact.

As challenging as all this was, I began to realize that the really hard part about quitting was being focused on not only my *feelings* but also on my *senses*. What do I mean by this? When you smoke a cigarette, all your senses are busy: you can see the cigarette and the smoke; taste and smell the smoke; listen to the striking of a match, the gentle crackling of the flame, the inhalation and exhalation; and feel the cigarette in your fingers. But suddenly, without the cigarette for "company," your senses are no longer occupied with some external stimulation. On top of this, you're also cut off from the physiologically calming and/or stimulating effects of the nicotine.

I became fascinated with this process. In fact, when I chose to no longer turn to smoking as a distraction or as a way to relax (as many of us do with food), my awareness of being with myself and my feelings heightened. What feelings had smoking helped me to handle? During the next few months (even years), I would have scores of opportunities to find out. Over time, I came to realize that I wanted to reach for a cigarette whenever I was experiencing strong emotions — either positive or negative. Was I stressed out? Depressed? Thrilled? Joyous? Regardless of the feeling, for months after I had stopped smoking, my initial instinct was to reach for a cigarette rather than to access my feelings and be willing to sit with them.

As with any addiction, I had been turning to cigarettes to avoid or to cut myself off from my feelings. Now, after years of not smoking, I realize that to be successful at quitting smoking permanently not only did I first need to identify my feelings each time a craving for a cigarette hit, but I also needed to allow myself to experience both positive and negative emotions. And then the hardest part (at first): to be alone in the moment with myself and my feelings — without seeking distraction from a cigarette and to make decisions about what to do with myself and my thoughts and feelings now that I'm not turning my attention to cigarettes as a distraction.

The same lessons also apply to food. Until you're willing to be alone with yourself and your feelings, food is more likely to control you, rather than you, it. Until you develop the ability both to find and identify your feelings before, during, and after eating, not only will you not experience your emotions, but you also won't be able to enjoy the moment or the emotional benefits in your meals fully. But there's still more to the challenge: if you're not filling your time with food and eating, thinking about food and eating, or trying to will yourself *not* to eat, what activities, thoughts, and people can you turn to instead of food?

Inside Out, Outside In

Accessing the healing secret of feelings calls for using your personal situation and feelings to decide what, how, how much, and whether to eat. Such an approach is the inverse of what most of us have learned about food and nutrition, which is to depend solely on external, objective, scientific information to determine our food choices. By now we know that the biological, scientific approach by itself won't lead to true, optimal eating and health (as discussed in the introduction). What will then? In this chapter, I'm suggesting that the solution lies in acting on insights gained from merging objective, scientific nutrition information with ancient, intuitive food-related wisdom. It's to this mix that you add your own internal "sensors" and feelings, which calls for being aware of your feelings before, during, and after eating, then fine-tuning your meals based on your own situation, needs, and feelings. In other words, it means eating from the inside out rather than from the outside in.

When you take the time to tune into your feelings on such a deep level, you open yourself up to creating a new dining experience that actually holds the power to transform a head-oriented relationship to food into a heartfelt, more satisfying connection. By creating a conscious awareness of your body/mind when you eat, you also become involved in, and aware of, the dynamic interaction of your food and your self. In turn, you empower each bite with fresh perceptions and the possibility of transforming both your feelings and the meaning and purpose of food in your life.

To Thine Own Self Be True

"Communication is the most important skill in life," writes Stephen Covey in *The 7 Habits of Highly Effective People*. In terms of food and feelings, this means that you may transform your relationship with food if you have open, honest communication between the feelings that guide you through life — whether they be "positive" (joy, serenity, love) or "negative" (regret, boredom, anger, hostility, judgment) — and the food you eat. As I noted earlier, developing optimal two-way communication between your feelings and your food is a two-step dance. The first step begins with your willingness to hear the "emotional music" in your meals. The second step calls for opening yourself to hearing the subtle notes that your mind/body play when you eat, to listening to the sounds and sensations that manifest throughout every stage of your meal.

How does this work in real life? To begin, ask yourself what's prompting you to eat: your hunger or your feelings? Continue checking in by deciding if you *feel* hungry, if you *feel* full, if you *feel* like having lettuce or lasagna. But I'm also proposing that you identify "emotional eating" feelings that sometimes signal or trigger you to eat — such as anxiety, loneliness, depression, fatigue, or fear — as well as positive, celebratory feelings, such as being happy, joyful, optimistic, or hopeful.

During the many years that I've counseled people, I've come to realize that the beliefs, thoughts, and feelings surrounding food have become a huge, often all-consuming problem for many of us. While I don't purport to have an easy solution to what is obviously a deeply rooted, multidimensional problem, I'm suggesting in this chapter that your potent feelings about food are not only the problem, they're also where the solution lies. In other words, you can use your feelings to become aware of the healing message in your meals. And the converse is also true: as you observe your feelings, you can turn to food to gain more control over your feelings, moods, and cravings. Such self-reflection is called "self-referral." In *Perfect Weight*, Deepak Chopra states that "in our society, self-referral is, unfortunately, very uncommon. It simply means looking inside yourself...to influence your thoughts or actions." He states that the alternative is: "object referral, whereby people respond to external cues that govern behavior."

From this perspective, following somebody else's prescription about what, how, and when to eat is a type of object referral. This includes following the latest fad diet or eating because the clock says you should. Not only do these strategies not work long-term, but they also encourage you to fill your time following, and thinking about, dietary rules and regulations instead of enjoying your life and your meals by eating what is optimal and enjoyable for you at any given moment. With Americans weighing in as the fattest people in the world — and with escalating food-linked ailments such as diabetes and high blood pressure — we have proven our object-referral approach to be ineffective; it's simply not working.

Often labeled "behavior modification" by therapists, the object-referral approach takes the form of such external suggestions as: put your fork down while chewing and between bites. Eat only when sitting down. Keep a food diary. Don't eat between meals. Eat small servings throughout the day. Or walk around the block instead of to the refrigerator. In other words, take stock of your food-related behavior and the foods you eat and then — based on this objective analysis — make changes or improvements in either what (Twinkies or turnips, for instance) or how (chewing thoroughly) you're eating.

As many of you know, with Americans' notorious failure rate at losing weight and keeping it off (fewer than 5 percent of us manage it), such concrete suggestions simply aren't working. Many of you also sense that object-referral advice isn't too appetizing, and that by following dietary dogma, your mind/body won't be truly satisfied. Realizing the limitations of the object-referral mentality, then-teenager Shauna Shamus commented, "I went on a diet for a month and lost thirty days of my life."

Self-referral — turning inward before, during, and after eating — is the opposite of the outward-directed object referral. Isn't it time to look closer at this approach, to explore what has worked for our ancestors for thousands of years? Isn't it time to reclaim your life, rather than to continue turning it over to food fallacies and fantasies and eating what you "should"? Isn't it time to acknowledge that the 95-plus percent failure rate of diets means that we're continuing to do something that isn't working? Isn't it time to ask different questions and to seek other solutions to our cravings, out-of-control binges, and food obsessions? In other words, if a successful relationship with food doesn't lie in external dietary dogma, where then does it lie? The answer is within yourself, in meeting the challenge of using your incredible human consciousness by tuning in to your feelings before, during, and after you eat.

Yoga's Food-Mood Message

Such an internal dance — with your awareness and feelings as partners — may seem strange, even difficult, at first. But be assured, you're in good company: most world religions and cultural traditions are steeped in dietary wisdom about food and feelings. For instance, five thousand years ago, ancient yogis (called *rishis*) created a food philosophy with feelings at its core. Especially in *anna* yoga (the yoga of food), devout yogis and Hindus learned to choose particular foods specifically because of their mind/body benefits, because of the way they affect the mind and emotions.

Swami Dharmananda, a spiritual teacher at the Adhyathma Sadhana Kendra Yoga Center in New Delhi, India, talked with me about the food-mood link espoused in the Bhagavad Gita, Hinduism's main scripture. We had an opportunity to talk when I visited New Delhi to present at a lifestyle conference. "In India we do not define food as you do in the West, meaning in terms of fat, protein, and carbohydrates. Instead, we classify food into three types (*gunas*, based on how they directly affect the mind." One category of yogic nutrition promotes a state of inertia, a lack of energy (*tamas*); on the other side is *rajas*, linked with an aggressive, overactive state; and *sattva* brings a balanced state of mind. According to the Bhagavad Gita, these three categories are attributes of nature that reflect your natural temperament and emotional moods. Based on this nutritional philosophy, the food you eat and the liquids you drink either enhance or diminish these qualities.

Which foods promote these various states of mind? *Sattvic* foods are natural, simple, and as close to their original state as possible. They include fruits, vegetables, grains, legumes (beans and peas), nuts and seeds, and dairy products, especially fresh milk and yogurt. These foods have been found not only to promote a calm, relaxed state in the *sattva*-natured person but are also believed to enhance health and happiness, a sense of cheerfulness, and a kind nature. In essence, these are the foods of the yogic diet.

On the other end of the spectrum, stimulating *rajas* foods and beverages — such as coffee, garlic, onions, and hot peppers — are thought to further energize an already high-energy, *rajas*-natured person. And a *tamas*-based diet — consisting of much high-fat animal-based foods, frozen food, processed food, pickled or preserved foods that are past their prime, and alcohol — is thought to contribute to laziness and a lack of alertness in the naturally low-key *tamas*-natured person.

The message is clear: yogis believe not only that food influences our emotions but also that each time we eat we have an opportunity to focus on, and connect with, our body/mind. Seen in this light, each food we choose to eat may be looked at as an opportunity not only to feed the body but also to fine-tune our moods and emotions.

Before, During, and After in Action

Let me show how eating both from and for your feelings recreates the kind of relationship with food and your body/mind that served our ancestors for millennia. A friend of mine named Nischala Devi is an international yoga master and author of *The Healing Path of Yoga;* before becoming a teacher and author, she was a swami for almost twenty years. My husband, Larry, and I spent a weekend in the country with Devi and her husband, Bhashkar, and shared many meals together. When I asked her to talk with me about how yogis relate to food through feelings and the senses, she was effusive. In hindsight, I realized she was really talking about being aware of food-related feelings before, during, and after eating.

🦋 *Before.* "A feeling of hunger is your body's built-in clock telling you it's time to eat," she explained. "When you're truly hungry, the desire to eat won't go away if you 'wait it out.'" In essence, during the years when she was a swami, Devi had cultivated the ability to tune in to how hungry she felt before eating and then to use that (self-referring) knowledge to make a decision about whether to eat. Devi told me that when she's ready to eat, she lets go of analytical, work-related issues that demand intense attention and/or personal problems that cause her concern or worry. Instead, for the time being — with the food in front of her — she moves into what I call "positive-feeling mode." This is based on the yogic belief that the mentality we bring to food — before, during, and after eating — is an important component of creating emotional well-being.

🦋 *During.* Devi's deep regard for the food-feeling connection continues throughout the meal. I watched as she and Bhashkar (also a practitioner of yoga) sometimes ate in silence. When I asked if this practice was intentional, I learned that the silence allowed them to intentionally savor the food. When conversation flowed, it was light and gay." This isn't a time to discuss income tax or a challenging work project," says Devi. "Because then you're feeling anxious while eating; your stomach reacts, your whole body reacts, and the food isn't metabolized well."

During the meal, Devi continued to draw her attention to how full she was feeling from minute to minute. Somewhat? Just right? Stuffed? (To help you identify how full you're feeling, yogic nutrition offers the following guideline: stop eating when three-quarters of the stomach is full. This is because ancient yogic scripture tells us that the stomach is about the size of your fist; therefore, filling your stomach about three-quarters during a meal leaves enough room for digestive enzymes to break down food.) Overeating — even balanced, healthful, plant-based *sattvic* foods — can render them unhealthful and *tamasic.*

🦋 *After.* When Devi recognizes she's had enough, she stops eating. As a matter of fact, she told me that once, having realized she was sated while having dinner in silence at the ashram (spiritual center) where she'd lived for years, she stopped eating in "mid-bite," then put the fork down.

When she's finished eating, she typically takes five or ten minutes to feel satisfied, calm, and appreciative of the meal. In other words, she continues to keep her feelings positive while savoring the food as it digests. Although taking the time to relax after a meal may be unusual in America, it's common in many parts of the world. It's an especially common experience for Devi, who gives seminars and workshops about yoga worldwide. "In India," she recalls, "even if you're with a group, your host will take you into a big room to lie down on the floor and rest after eating. This would be considered a strange thing to do in the United States, but if you think about it, it's a way to feel relaxed and to respect your body/mind." Do yogis believe there are health benefits to be gained by remaining calm and peaceful after you've had a meal? Absolutely. "When you feel calm after eating," offers Devi, "it's easier for your body to assimilate what you've eaten."

Reuniting Mind and Matter

As you can see, the yogic nutrition philosophy is a time-honored tradition steeped in dietary wisdom about food and feelings. However, this ageless regard for the symbiotic connection between food and its effects on the mind/body may not be familiar to many of you. This is because the mind/body link gradually became obscured in Western thinking when the French philosopher and mathematician René Descartes (1596–1650) speculated that the mind (the conscious self that's aware of feelings, thought, and actions) and the body (or matter in general) were separate and distinct entities. As a rationalist, Descartes believed that all knowledge of the world is ultimately derived from pure reason, that is, from innate and self-evident truths with no need of input from the senses. On the opposite end of the spectrum, the philosophy of Empiricism held that all knowledge is ultimately derived from the senses.

Over the centuries, Western culture came to play out both sides of this mind/body split. On the one hand, the Western scientific perspective, which has evolved since Descartes, accepts that our feelings and consciousness are completely dependent on matter and the body; on the other extreme, it sees the mind as being completely independent of the senses, body chemistry, and food (creating a one-way relationship). But, as the adage goes, if you wait long enough, what's been out of fashion comes into vogue again. This is certainly true for the link between food and feelings. During the latter part of the twentieth century (about four centuries after Descartes separated mind and matter), researchers began to focus their technology on the body-mind bridge and the way in which food affects feelings.

The Emotional Messengers in Food

Today, the focus is back on interdependence of the body/mind, and food and feelings are, once again, being intimately linked. Some call this new focus food-mood research. Others call it nutritional neuroscience. Still others link it to mind/body medicine and eating disorders. The Bhagavad Gita frames it around the three *guna*s. I call it psychological nutrition. However it's labeled, modern science is discovering that foods release substances in our bodies that affect our moods and, conversely, that our moods often influence our food choices.

Ultimately, food-mood research is an investigation of food and the mind/body working together. This new field of nutrition began in the 1970s, when pioneering researchers Richard Wurtman, M.D., and Judith Wurtman, Ph.D., first linked food with mood when they found that the sugar and starch in carbohydrates (especially those found in fruits, vegetables, and grains) boosted a powerful brain chemical called serotonin. Soon they linked serotonin and other neurotransmitters (substances that pass information from cell to cell in the brain) to our every mood, emotion, or craving. For instance, they noted that eating carbohydrate-rich foods, such as potatoes or bread, elevated serotonin levels, which help you to feel more relaxed and calm. On the other hand, high-protein food, such as nonfat dairy and lean fish and poultry, had the opposite effect: these foods release substances that let you think and react more quickly and feel more alert and energetic.

How might modern nutrition neuroscience describe the post-meal sense of relaxation that Devi experienced after eating a *sattva*, plant- and carbohydrate-based meal? By taking the time to be aware of your feelings after you eat, you're setting the stage to allow the serotonin to "communicate" with you, which takes some fifteen or twenty minutes to register after you've consumed carbohydrates.

Apparently, carbohydrate-dense foods work their wonders first by providing a glucose response that releases the hormone insulin from the pancreas. In turn, the insulin triggers the absorption of amino acids (the building blocks of protein, of which there are twenty-two) from the bloodstream into the cells — all except one: tryptophan. Unopposed and circulating into the bloodstream at relatively high levels, tryptophan floods the brain and is converted into soothing serotonin. And when this alchemical interaction occurs, your mood improves.

"I'd Kill for a Cookie"

Other studies by researchers at Rockefeller University in New York point to cravings for carbohydrates as Mother Nature's way of informing us about what we need to eat to feel better. For women this could mean that the sugar and carbohydrate cravings many experience are a response to estrogen's effect on brain chemicals and blood-sugar levels.

To find out more about this, I talked with Catherine Christie, nutritionist and author of *I'd Kill for a Cookie*. "When estrogen levels fall and progesterone levels are high, serotonin levels drop," clarifies Dr. Christie. And because adequate levels of serotonin help us feel calm and relaxed, when levels become too low — especially during certain times of the menstrual cycle or during menopause — our appetite increases, along with carbohydrate cravings, potential overeating, and possible ensuing weight gain.

Unfortunately, to regulate and calm jumpy nerves, anger, and tension quickly, instead of turning to healthful potatoes or gravitating toward whole grains (discussed in detail in chapter 7) women, especially, often choose sugar-laden, highly processed (albeit carbohydrate-dense) fast foods to feel better. Some all-too-familiar examples are donuts, cookies, carrot cake, bread, corn chips, candy bars, or "liquid candy," commonly called soft drinks. But these foods may be defeating your purpose: Wurtman believes that the slowly digested, high-fat content of such foods inhibits production of serotonin. The end result is that instead of feeling soothed, you may feel sluggish, even drugged.

Such subtle mood switch-overs happen without your having to think about them. Keep in mind, though, that food-mood research is still in its infancy. While most researchers agree that a physiological change happens when we eat certain foods, not all agree on which comes first — food or mood. Because the chemical cornucopia in our brains and bodies is complex, it's hard to always establish a direct link between our brain chemistry and emotional response.

This situation is further complicated when you consider that you may have a predisposition for craving, say, chocolate chip cookies, because your mother rewarded you with them for doing well in school. Or perhaps choosing certain foods may not be about mood but about what your body must have to meet its nutritional needs; this may mean that you choose to snack on an orange for its vitamin-C content, not for its effect on your mood. Or perhaps eating a piece of pie may alleviate boredom; crunching hard and fast on chips, carrots, or celery could alleviate anger.

Designing Moods

When accessing the healing secret of feelings, the source of the information (ancient wisdom or modern science) isn't the key consideration for reaping the rewards; rather, it's the immediacy and awareness of the feelings that you bring to food — and that food brings to you — before, during, and after eating. As you enter into this internal dance with your body/mind, and are willing to experience your emotions and moods, to allow yourself simply to *be* with them, you are positioning yourself to transform meals into an opportunity for emotional growth and deep satisfaction.

The following is a primer of practical exercises and insights that show you how to access and experience the influence of food on feelings, and vice versa, the interplay between your feelings and food choices. As you begin to hear the emotion-rich notes in your food, you'll be empowered to create and orchestrate your own, personal, food-feeling symphony each time you eat.

⚜ *Calm down with carbohydrates.* Carbohydrate-based foods calm and relax you. Which foods are carbohydrate rich? The plant-based foods groups: grains (oats, rice, wheat, barley, rye), vegetables (especially potatoes), fruit (including bananas, cherries, pears), legumes (beans and peas), nuts and seeds; also milk. These foods — as well as refined sugar — encourage you to feel calm and relaxed because they release the naturally occurring chemical messenger serotonin. Carbohydrate-dense foods may also help you to sleep more soundly. How much is enough to reap the benefits? A single slice of bread, a small cracker, a teaspoon of honey, or a spoonful of cereal will activate soothing serotonin about twenty minutes after you've eaten.

⚜ *Perk up with protein.* Suppose that rather than seeking to be soothed, you want to feel alert and energized. When this is your motive, turn to protein-dense, low-fat foods — such as nonfat dairy products, lean fish or poultry, and high-protein legumes, especially soybeans. While the soothing-serotonin story includes carbohydrates, the amino acid tryptophan, and then serotonin production (discussed in detail earlier in the chapter), the perky-protein trilogy starts with a high-protein food that triggers the production of the amino acid tyrosine; in turn, the chemical messengers norepinephrine and dopamine are released. The end result is that your mental acuity is enhanced.

Here are some perk-up possibilities: if you're feeling sluggish in the afternoon, try some nonfat yogurt (one cup is all it takes), a taste of water-packed tuna (perhaps about one or two tablespoons), or a sip of some fat-free soy milk. The key concept in enhancing mental acuity is to choose lean protein-based foods that contain as little fat as possible.

❦ *Figure the fat.* Not all fats are created equal. Some influence your feelings positively, others negatively.

❦ *"Smart" fats.* We've all heard that fish is "brain food" that makes you smarter. Well, it's true. The benefit to your brain comes from relatively high levels of essential fatty acids (EFAs) in fish, called linolenic acid (omega-3s, or n-3) and linoleic acid (omega-6, or n-6). These smart fats are also found in high concentrations in flax seeds (grind them up to increase absorption), soybeans, and walnuts.

❦ *Memory-dimming fat.* While EFAs may be considered smart fats, if you eat a diet high in saturated, hard fat, you're courting poor performance. Saturated fat is abundant in foods such as marbled meat; processed sausage, salami, and ham; and in dairy products such as whole milk, cheese, butter, and ice cream. Not only do diets high in "sat-fats" make you feel sluggish (by lowering the amount of circulating oxygen in your blood), they may also alter your mood by encouraging depression and perhaps impair memory. Unfortunately these sat-fats are common in the typical American diet (discussed in detail in chapter 7).

❦ *Beat the blues with B's.*Carbohydrates, protein, and fat are the major macronutrients that affect feelings. But food is also replete with micronutrients, such as vitamins and minerals, that also influence the way you feel. Some of the ultimate food-mood nutrients are members of the B vitamin family, which includes B1 (thiamine), B2 (riboflavin), B3 (niacin), B5 (pantothenic acid), B6 (pyridoxine), B7 (biotin), folic acid (also folacin or folate), and B12 (cobalamin). From diminishing depression to enhancing mental agility, the B vitamins can help. Following are some "B healthy" hints:

❦ *Get whole.* Whole grains (such as millet, barley, buckwheat, brown rice, whole wheat, and oats) can be beneficial blues busters, because the germ in whole grains is the key container of the B's. To ensure that a grain is whole and B-vitamin rich, read the label. If you do not see the word *whole* (as in whole wheat, whole oats, and so on), then the germ (and much of the fiber) is likely to be missing. Some B-smart suggestions: Buy brown rice instead of white. Choose whole-wheat bread in lieu of wheat (white) bread. Have a multigrain cereal for breakfast — either cold or cooked.

❧ **Shun sugar.** Of little nutritional value, refined white sugar damages and destroys B vitamins in the body, so consuming too much may contribute to deficiencies. The end result is possible depression. One theory about why sugar contributes to depression is that when you consume lots of sugar — which is abundant in processed foods such as muffins, candy, cookies, cake, ice cream, and soda — blood sugar (glucose) rises, along with endorphins (naturally occurring chemicals that contribute to a sense of relaxation and feelings of euphoria). But once sugar is metabolized, blood sugar levels plummet, along with endorphins. The end result is a "crash" that could contribute to depression and fatigue.

❧ **Avoid alcohol, cut caffeine.** Not only does consuming lots of sugary foods contribute to depression and fatigue by depleting the B vitamins, drinking too many caffeinated liquids (such as coffee and Coca-Cola) and alcoholic drinks (such liquor, wine, and beer) have a comparable influence, because consuming too much of these beverages reduces absorption of certain B vitamins. Deficiencies of vitamins B3 and B6 especially can contribute to bringing you down.

❧ **B-vitamin mood Rx.** Here are some examples of B3- and B6-rich foods that may bust the blues and bolster well-being:

B3: cooked beans and peas, peanuts and peanut butter, green peas, potatoes, whole grains, brewer's yeast (nutritional), milk

B6: wheat germ, soy beans, cooked beans and peas, peanuts, bananas, avocados, cabbage, cauliflower, potatoes, whole grain breads and cereals, dried fruit, collard greens, brown rice, walnuts

❧ **Choose chocolate (sometimes).** The enticing combination of creamy fat and sweet sugar (called "the dynamic duo" by dietitian and author Elizabeth Somer) may be a major reason why so many of us crave chocolate. Not only do chocolate and sugar release relaxing serotonin, the blues-busting benefits of endorphins that are liberated after consuming chocolate may be another reason why many of us crave this delicious, feel-good elixir. Surprisingly, it only takes a small amount of chocolate (one or two pieces, for instance) to access its elevating effects. Or savor and stretch the mood-enhancing benefits by lingering over a cup of low-fat, sugar-free hot cocoa; add just a teaspoon or two of sugar to enhance the flavor.

Recipes for Feeling

The above suggestions for designing your moods through food are but a sprinkling of possibilities for bringing on good feelings through what you eat. What follows are a few personal experiences I've had creating what I call "feeling recipes." One evolved serendipitously when I least expected to reap the rewards of the impact of my meal on my mood; the others are seasonal ingredients that illuminate the incredible influence that feelings may have on the foods we choose throughout the year.

Instant Gratification

Routine. Comfort. Familiarity. That's what's on my morning menu most of the time. But on one memorable morning when I broke with tradition, I inadvertently experienced an unforgettable lesson about the power of food over feelings.

Most of us tend to choose the same types of food each day, such as some toast or cereal for breakfast, a sandwich or salad for lunch, and perhaps fish, chicken, or pasta as a main course for dinner. For me, a typical breakfast includes a small fruit smoothie and multigrain cereal moistened with nonfat soy milk. Often I add garnishes that include a sprinkling of ground flaxseed, oat or wheat bran, and a tablespoon of brown sugar. After eating, I often seek serenity with a cup of green tea. Not only does it stir my spirit, but tea also seems to open my mind to musings and memories.

One morning, not only did I deviate from my breakfast routine, I skipped it completely. Leaving early to work out at my local health club, my only nourishment had been a glass of orange juice. After exercising, I instantly went into "chore mode" instead of going home to have breakfast. Then, not surprisingly, about an hour after I'd left the health club, I felt overwhelmingly, ravenously hungry. But not wanting to break stride with my tasks — with which I was almost finished — I dashed into a local café and ordered a chai soy latte (a concoction of spiced black tea, foamy soy milk, and honey). My intention was to assuage my hunger until I could get home to eat a more complete, healthful breakfast.

Leaving the café, I began the final chore: to mail an important document at my local post office. With about five people ahead of me in line, I thought my wait would be short. But I was wrong. Rather, each customer seemed to have complicated tasks to perform. After I'd waited for fifteen minutes, not only was the line still five-people long, the same three customers were still at the same mail stations. Time seemed to have stopped.

During these frustrating minutes, I reminded myself that the reward of patience is patience (ancient Chinese wisdom), but I was feeling far from patient; rather, I was growing increasingly cranky and bored. And then, with no intentional effort on my part, in an instant, I suddenly felt calm, relaxed, and happy, even euphoric. Amazed at my immediate change of mood, I realized that nature had turned on the serotonin switch in my mind/body via the carbohydrate- and caffeine-laden chai soy latte I'd consumed not too long ago. Unintentionally, I had conducted a food-mood experiment on myself, which revealed that food does, indeed, affect mood...if we allow ourselves to listen to the invisible messages that emerge from what we consume.

The Seasons and Food

The healing secret of feelings frequently focuses on emotions that food may release, but the inverse is also true: your feelings and moods may influence the foods you choose — especially throughout the seasons. When you expand your enjoyment of food by linking your feelings to the moods of fall, winter, spring, and summer, your awareness can work like a light that illuminates the subtle sensations and pleasures that are waiting to be revealed when you eat.

❧ *Fall.* For as long as I can remember, I've longed to be in New England during the fall. As the air becomes brisk and the scent of smoke from fireplaces fills the air, the leaves burst with a range of vibrant golden and amber tones that mimic the sunset. For me, the tones of autumn reflect the transition from the heat of summer to the still, grayness of winter — just as the glow of dying embers serves as a bridge from vibrant, hot flames to pallid, pale ash.

When I'm surrounded by the bittersweet mood of autumn, I often marvel at the way the colors of this season materialize in food: the deep orange of pumpkin, the golden richness of acorn squash, the earthy brown of chestnuts. Intent on ingesting these marvelous manifestations of fall, I often create some squash soup on the spot. The key ingredients include steamed squash, roasted chestnuts, some fresh tarragon, and chopped scallions. The supporting cast: a mere tablespoon of extra-virgin olive oil; salt and freshly ground pepper, to taste; a bit of brown sugar; and grated fresh ginger — all blended together, then simmered slowly in a miso-based broth.

As I garnish the golden soup with a flicker of freshly grated nutmeg, I savor each spoonful and the way in which the soup makes me feel both grounded and connected to the richness of the earth and the change in seasons. Then, unexpectedly, I feel more than just nourished by the soup; my soul is somehow illuminated by its amber radiance.

❧ *Winter.* It is early in the evening. Larry and I are sitting in a restaurant in Müren, Switzerland, relishing the respite from the icy chill of the snowy winter landscape outside. We are vacationing, taking a break from the research we're doing with heart patients at medical centers in both Germany and Holland. To get to this resort town, we took a slow, squeaky tram up the side of a steep, snowy mountain. Because Müren is so high up and hard to reach, there are no cars there. Instead, the busyness of everyday life is replaced with a special sense of solitude and serenity, and in winter, with the opaque, flat, silent quality that comes with snow. Scanning the menu, we're feeling as if we're perched on top of the world in a winter wonderland.

Because of the locale and season, I am feeling a subtle sense of withdrawal from the world; it is a time of turning inward. With these winter-inspired feelings in my heart, some of my most unforgettable food feelings emerged. To be truthful, I don't remember much about what we ate that first night in Müren. But I do recall — vividly — the feelings, mood, and atmosphere that flavored my dining experience: the soothing serenity of hushed conversation, the cozy comfort of being surrounded by steamed-up windows, the flicker of candlelight on each table, the soothing influence of the scents emanating from the kitchen, and the welcoming warmth of the food we ate. Blended together, all these mood-enhancing ingredients created a particular internal ambience in my soul as I ate — one that provided a perfect antidote to the icy cold and utter blackness of the moonless winter night that waited for us outside.

❧ *Summer.* There's a sunnier side to Switzerland: summertime, summer showers, and impromptu meals spiced with friendship and appreciation for an improvised menu. During yet another sojourn in Switzerland — this time during the summer — Larry and I took a day-long hike to Scoul, a romantic town in eastern Switzerland; our longtime friend and colleague, Stephen Sparler, joined us.

After eight hours of hiking in the countryside and journeying from village to village, Scoul was an especially welcome site. Situated in a valley between two mountain ranges, peppered with bumpy cobblestoned streets, and dotted with handmade murals on buildings, its many charms made navigating the multitude of switchbacks that led down into this village well worth the effort. A sudden summer shower added to the charm, as did the furnished atelier-style apartment we found — replete with a well-equipped kitchen — and a nearby local grocery store where we purchased food for dinner. Ah, the spirit of summer! We were pleasantly tired from our long hike, drenched from the sudden downpour, and glowing from a day spent outdoors hiking in the sunshine. It had been a nature-filled day, full of vast vistas, winding hiking trails, and the fragrant scents of summer. I was happy to the point of giddiness, sunlit from the inside, sated by the rain, and whole-heartedly hungry from the hike. In this state of mind, I prepared a simple dinner in our quaint kitchen. While Larry and Stephen went for a beer in a nearby tavern, I boiled some simple spaghetti, warmed and stirred the spicy, herb-filled tomato sauce, washed and chopped lettuce, carrots, and cucumbers for the salad, sliced the loaf of crusty bread purchased from the bakery just next door, and poured the red wine. The food was as casual, cozy, and sponta-neous as my mood.

When they returned, the sun had set and it was dusk. I lit some candles, then served the steaming pasta and side dishes. Feeling relaxed and content, we sat around the table talking and remi-niscing about the day. As we talked and dined on the impromptu meal, I glanced outside the kitchen's angled attic window in time to see some stars sparkling in Switzerland's summertime night sky.

❧ *Spring.* During a springtime trip to my local farmers' mar-ket, I learned that flowers — edible flowers, that is — can be part of a palate-pleasing feast. Early one morning while I was selecting some fresh organic salad greens, my eyes lit on two colorful bins: one filled with rose petals, the other with squash blossoms. Fascinated by the idea of being able to consume — literally — these universal manifestations of springtime, I bought a bagful of each. When I got home, I reflected on the flowers and the feelings and thoughts that often bloom in spring: a sense of hope and optimism, a tug toward new beginnings, and reflections on birth and rebirth.

Feeling joyful and playful, I considered making some rose-petal jam, but I was on deadline with a project and didn't have the time. What I could accomplish, though, was to enhance and ingest the spirit of springtime by using pretty, fragrant rose petals as a garnish for some sorbet. Though I knew the petals were pesticide free, I still washed them gently in a bowl of warm water. I then shook some dry, while I used the moisture on the remaining rose petals to attract and hold the confectioners' sugar in which I dipped them.

Throughout the week, I celebrated spring each time I snacked on some petals — with or without sorbet. And each time I noticed one of the golden yellow squash blooms that I had blended into the mixed salad, or reflected on the red rose petals that lingered — ever so delicately — near the raspberry sorbet (my favorite), my heart smiled at the promise of new life and the bloom of new beginnings that spring brings.

chapter four

The Healing Secret of Mindfulness

Bring moment-to-moment nonjudgmental
awareness to each aspect of the meal.

The extent to which our food reveals itself depends on
us.... Contemplating our food for a few seconds before eating,
and eating in mindfulness, can bring us much happiness.

— *Thich Nhat Hanh,* Peace in Every Step

With the healing secret of mindfulness, I am introducing you to the first of three spiritual nutrition healing secrets that will enrich and nourish both your food experience and your soul. The other two, appreciation and connection, will be discussed in detail in the following chapters. When you hold these three simple but profound healing secrets in your heart while preparing food, cooking, eating, digesting — even while cleaning up after a meal — both you and the health-enhancing flavors in your food will flourish.

The healing secret of mindfulness helps you bring moment-to-moment nonjudgmental awareness to each aspect of your meal. Within the context of mindfulness, spirituality means intermingling your consciousness with the mystery of life (Higher Power, God, Supreme Being) inherent in food by remaining aware that food is life giving and life containing, as are we human beings. Each of the three chapters about spiritual nutrition will show you how to integrate and mix these spiritual ingredients into your meals — carefully, consciously, and completely.

Soul Food

Mindfulness is about more than having the intention to be aware; it is also pure awareness in that it calls for "being aware of being aware." In science, a meta-analysis is research of other studies on a particular subject. The healing secret of mindfulness can be called a "meta-secret" that reinforces all the other healing secrets discussed throughout this book. For instance, socially, mindfulness enhances the experience of dining and sharing food with others. When applied to feelings, mindfulness provides insights into food-related feelings, even how your feelings influence digestion. Physically, it empowers you to choose health-enhancing foods. And spiritually, it holds the power to heal your soul. How so? When I talked with mindfulness and stress-management expert Jon Kabat-Zinn, he shared this exceptional insight: "Mindfulness meditation is actually a process of nourishment, an oxygen line straight into the soul. It's the universe expressing through you, making it an aspect of the sacred."

How does the "oxygen line" of mindfulness heal the soul? Consider how a magnifying glass can focus the sun's rays. If you take a magnifying glass out into the sunlight and hold it so that it catches the rays directly, it will concentrate the light into such an intense point of light that it can actually burn a hole through paper. Mindfulness works the same way. When you gather your thoughts and focus your attention on one point of thought, action, or the food before you, you ignite insight, wisdom, and healing energy. In this way, your one-pointed attention to each aspect of the meal allows you to meet and therefore heal the deepest parts of your being.

The Mindful "Fruit Route"

To glean the benefits of infusing nonjudgmental mindfulness into meals, it's key for you to realize that this healing secret is relevant to more than formal meals or to specific social occasions. Let me demonstrate how cultivating food-linked mindfulness may be applied to almost any food-oriented circumstance, how being mindful can turn an everyday activity into an extraordinary, transformative journey.

For quite a long time, my husband, Larry, worked in the small coastal town in northern California where we live. Because the distance from home to work was fairly short, much of the time he'd ride his bicycle to the office, enjoying the views from the hillside above the bay and the winding, narrow streets. But he especially relished the abundance of fruit trees scattered throughout the public paths. After a while, he started referring to his commute as his "fruit route." Through ongoing observation and by paying attention to nature's details, Larry got to know where each type of fruit tree was located and when it would ripen. For instance, the plum trees in a nearby shady grove would be the first to ripen in the spring. The apricot tree near the local library would be next. Wild blackberry bushes would flourish in the summer. In late summer, Larry discovered ripe peaches not too far from his office. And by winter, when all the other fruit trees would be finished for the year, the orange tree would just begin to bear its fruit.

"After traveling this fruit route for a year," he told me, "I came to know the growing cycle of each tree, when they would begin to bloom, and later how weighted some trees were by their fruit." Over a period of three months, he watched as a peach would turn from a small green ball into a golden yellow, ripe fruit. And then the fruit would become overly ripe and start to fall and drop off.

He especially watched the plum trees. Because they were the first to bloom in the spring, he'd anticipate seeing this signal that spring would soon follow. In the early morning hours, Larry would often rest his bicycle against a bush so that he could sample some plums from three or four of his favorite trees. Because he'd observed the trees' source of water and available sunlight, he came to know which ones would produce the best fruit. And knowing that the sunlight made certain plums sweeter than those that grew in the shade, he selected the ripest red, green, or yellow plums from the sunny side of the tree. If the plums or other fruit were especially tasty, he'd pick more and take them to work to share with colleagues.

Larry summed up both his short- and long-term observations of his odyssey this way: "By focusing my senses on the fruit while eating it, I brought moment-to-moment awareness to the immediate experience of eating. But by observing both the trees and the fruit throughout the seasons, I was being mindful in yet another way: I remained aware of the longer cycles that nature creates, those invisible, transitory moments that make up not only our meals, but our life."

Paths to Mindfulness

The spiritual dimension of mindfulness was born in meditation, a practice that reaches back thousands of years. When you bring mindful awareness to each aspect of your meals, you're actually participating in the ancient practice of meditation, described by religious historian Mircea Eliade as "deep, continued reflection, a concentrated dwelling in thought." There's another dimension to mindfulness, though. It also implies that you're aware of your awareness, of your choice to focus on food and food-related activities.

Cultivating mindfulness — what Kabat-Zinn describes as "paying attention intentionally" — is rooted in many ancient traditions, especially Buddhism. One of Buddhism's earliest sutras (scriptures), called the Mindfulness Sutra, provides actual guidelines for cultivating moment-to-moment awareness that is judgment free and impartial, a focus that encourages awakening to the detail of each moment. Such attention to detail is inherent in the way devout Buddhists relate to all aspects of life — including food and beverages. For instance, with roots in Buddhism, Japan's Way of Tea (*Chado*) — referred to in the West as the Japanese Tea Ceremony (*Chanoyu*) — turns the simple act of infusing boiling water with tea leaves into a timeless ritual of aestheticism that encourages mindfulness through what author and Japanese tea master Kakuzo

Okakura describes as "listening to the unspoken, gazing upon the unseen."

Indeed, the pleasure derived from the ceremony lies in paying attention to the moment-to-moment unfolding of its subtle notes: the pouring of water, the clink of the lid on the iron teakettle, or the whisking of the powdered green tea as it's turned into a light, frothy brew. The next moment may present the flat tone of placing the tea bowl on the mat, the ongoing, varied cadences of conversation, or the silences between the notes. Through such moment-to-moment mindfulness, the connection and relationship among ourselves, the tea, the tearoom, and others, unfolds.

Like Buddhists, yogis also espouse meditating mindfully to pursue connection with the Divine. Taoists turn to meditation as a way to harmonize with everything and all moments. The Jewish mystical teaching of the Kabbalah encourages meditation (watchfulness) to transport consciousness through what it describes as "gateways." Early Christian monks and saints practiced meditation as a stringent contemplative process to achieve spiritual exaltation. And Islam's mystical Sufis dance meditatively to suffuse their minds, hearts, and souls with the Absolute. No matter how diverse these practices may seem, the underlying intention is the same: making the conscious decision to switch from an aimless or diffused awareness to a mindful way of being in the world — as when we partake of the tea ceremony or prepare and eat a meal.

The Nonjudgmental Dimension

If the spiritual dimension of mindfulness was born in meditation, its nonjudgmental element evolved from Buddhist beliefs that encourage detachment: observing and noticing feelings, thoughts, or opinions about food and eating and all activities as they arise, and then letting them go. This practice calls for recognizing that thoughts and feelings are transient and that they have nothing to do with the food in front of you.

If you're to reap the emotional and physical benefits of mindfulness, letting go of judging yourself, others, and food is one key to your success. Letting go is no easy feat, though, because it's all too easy to get sidetracked by judgmental thinking. Entering into a judgmental frame of mind is an alluring way to deal with issues, to sort, to control, to ponder. Because of its nature, being judgmental provides a sustained path of attention, which holds the power to carry you completely away from mindfully observing — and releasing — the flow of mental activity. With judgment, you quickly get lost in your train of thought rather than *observing* the train of thought (being aware of being aware). When this happens, you're out of the moment.

With food, many of us use judgment to assign all kinds of (mostly) negative values to ourselves, to others, and to the food itself. We carry on constant, internal, judgment-filled chatter that we often take for granted:

"I was really good today," we say when we've eaten what we think we should.

"Oh, I gave into my craving and ate that *sinful* chocolate cake; I feel so guilty."

"You don't look well. Have you lost weight?" we might say to a friend.

"I know I should become a vegetarian, but I don't want to look like one" (yes, I actually overheard this comment).

And then, of course, there's judging what others eat or what we think others should eat (less fat, more fat, less carbohydrates, more protein, and so on). Many of us also carry on internal dialogues, concerned that others will judge us as gluttonous if we take second servings or if we order what we really want (so we select a salad when we're out with friends, then eat what we really want when we get home).

Still others place moral judgment on whether it's acceptable to consume animal-based food, such as beef, chicken, fish, and even dairy products. But is such a fundamentalist approach to food typical of our spiritual heritage? Not according to the tenets of Buddhism. Although meat isn't explicitly forbidden in some Buddhist traditions, a vow against killing is interpreted by many to include avoiding the ingestion of animal-based food. But Tibetans and other Buddhists sometimes eat meat — with the concession of minimizing the taking of life as much as possible (for instance, taking the life of one cow, instead of the life of four thousand shrimp). Along with this goes the practice of not judging others' eating of meat as being "bad."

When I had the pleasure of talking with chef, Buddhist teacher, and author Edward Espe Brown, I discovered more about Buddhism's time-honored tradition of withholding judgment about eating meat. "It's their version of going back to the Bud-dhist practice of [monks] receiving food that is offered to them [by others]," he said. "You don't try to make others wrong by saying 'I don't eat that.' This means not trying to convince others that they should eat the way you do — and then putting them in [nutrition] jail if they eat what you think are 'wrong' foods."

The Pitfalls of Impatience

Along with being judgmental, another deterrent to mindfulness is worth considering: what I call hurry sickness. As you pursue creating meals mindfully, you'll find that being in a hurry is just as destructive to being in the moment as being judgmental is. When you're impatient, you're actually trying to live in the future, since you're in a hurry to not be where you are at present. But you pay a price when your impatience takes you out of the here and now: resent the time it takes to chop some vegetables, and you may cut yourself; toss some food into the fridge and you may spill it; leave the stove to do something else, or speed up the cooking process by turning up the flame too high, and the food is likely to burn.

Not only is your food likely to suffer, but when you eat quickly, you may end up with an upset stomach, not really tasting the food, and a sense of lingering, unsatisfied hunger. If you diffuse your consciousness further by task-stacking (talking on the phone while cooking, working at the computer or watching TV while eating), then true mindfulness becomes even more elusive.

Metabolizing Mindfulness

The health benefits of switching from mindless eating to creating meals mindfully are well worth the effort. When you let go of feelings and thoughts as they arise and keep your attention focused on your food, you're opening yourself to one of the healing messages inherent in mindfulness: altering, and taking advantage of, the way you metabolize food.

A brilliant suggestion that mindfulness is beneficial to digestion was revealed when researcher Donald Morse, M.D., professor emeritus at Temple University in Philadelphia, and colleagues, studied the impact on digestion when eating mindfully as opposed to eating while distracted and stressed. In Morse's study, a group of women college students meditated for five minutes before eating cereal; another group performed mental arithmetic (as a form of distraction and stress) for five minutes before eating the cereal. Afterward, Dr. Morse and his team measured the saliva of each group. Amazingly, those who meditated mindfully before eating produced 22 percent more of the digestive enzyme alpha-amylase. Not only is alpha-amylase important because it helps you digest B vitamins, it also increases the metabolism of carbohydrate-dense foods, such as cereal, pasta, and bread.

Of course, the design of the study poses an unanswered question, Did meditating before eating increase alpha-amylase, or did doing math before eating decrease it? A third group — one in which students ate in a relaxed (but not meditative) frame of mind might have answered this question. But for now, this study raises the possibility that if you eat while distracted or stressed (without mindfulness), you're likely to absorb fewer nutrients than your body needs to function optimally. It also "shows that there's a real benefit to having a leisurely meal," said Dr. Morse in *American Health* magazine. "The decrease in alpha-amylase production is just the tip of the iceberg. When you gulp down your food, your entire digestive system is affected."

Another hint that eating mindfully enhances digestion surfaced when researcher L. W. McCuaig studied the saliva of a male meditator over a six-month period. Instead of targeting enzymes in saliva, McCuaig focused on the minerals. He found that meditation increased salivary minerals, all of which are important to optimal digestion. Increases ranged from magnesium (42 percent) and calcium (36 percent) to potassium (23 percent) and sodium (70 percent); the protein content of the saliva also increased by 60 percent. Interestingly, a mere ten minutes after meditation, the levels of these nutrients in saliva had already decreased. Because McCuaig's study was done with one person, we don't know how others would respond. Even so, his research also raises the possibility that practicing focused awareness while eating increases our production of nutrients.

The more I reflect on mindfulness, the more I'm convinced that a mystical interconnection and healing magic occur when we focus our attention while eating. As these studies suggest, when we pay attention to our food and eat with meditative awareness, our body responds by producing nutrients that may help to metabolize food. In this way, the power of awareness facilitates both health and healing.

"Type A" and "Type B" Behavior

"The quality of one's life depends on the quality of attention," writes Deepak Chopra in *Ageless Body, Timeless Mind*. So, too, does the quality of one's health. Not only may it affect your peace of mind, digestion, and the absorption of nutrients, eating with a distracted, agitated consciousness has other health-threatening implications: by influencing the way in which you metabolize fat, it may affect your chances of developing heart disease.

Let me explain the groundbreaking study that revealed such amazing ideas. In the mid-1960s, pioneering cardiologists Drs. Meyer Friedman and Ray Rosenman coined the phrase "Type A behavior" to describe the pattern of "hurry sickness" and free-floating hostility that they observed in many of their heart patients. Interestingly, one of the key observations that led to their discovery came from a local upholsterer. While working on Dr. Friedman's waiting room chairs, the upholsterer noticed that the chairs were heavily worn at the front of the seat and arms, something not typical in other doctors' offices where he had worked. This stark reminder of heart patients' (nonmindful) impatience helped to inspire Friedman and Rosenman to look more closely at their patients' behavior, which led to their ideas about Type A behavior.

On closer scrutiny, Friedman and Rosenman also found these patients to be easily angered, self-centered, ambitious, competitive, and perfectionistic. When these Type A patients talked, their speech was emphatic and quick, they interrupted often, and they were fidgety, restless, and judgmental (all attributes that are the antithesis of mindfulness). And when they were asked, Do you like to linger at the table when eating, or do you prefer to get up and go? the Type A's consistently preferred to "get up and go."

Friedman and Rosenman coined the term "Type B" to describe those who didn't display these traits. As a contrast, Type B's were calm, relaxed, easygoing, and patient (more likely to be mindful), with a high threshold for anger. Rather than interrupting, they listened carefully, were thoughtful when answering questions, and were nonjudgmental.

The "Sludging" Factor

After years of pioneering discoveries that linked Type A behavior to higher cholesterol levels and increased risk for heart attack, Dr. Friedman made yet another amazing discovery: the more patient, relaxed, nonjudgmental Type B's metabolized fat in food more effectively (and possibly, in a more heart-healthy way). Conversely, being Type A — living in a hard-driving, competitive, and impatient state of mind — significantly impaired the metabolism of fat. The end result was an increased risk of having a heart attack.

Such intriguing results surfaced after both Type A's and Type B's ingested a super-high fat snack consisting of a milk shake (whole milk, half-and-half, cream, two whole eggs, and ice cream) and two pats of butter on four shortbread cookies. One hour later, when Freidman and colleagues magnified photographs of the tiny vessels in the whites of the participants' eyes, they could actually see the capillaries of Type A's becoming clogged. Like too many logs impeding the flow of a river, the blood platelets and chylomicrons (the fat-carrying "basket" in blood) massed together to slow the blood flow. Dr. Friedman and colleagues coined the term *sludging* to describe this impaired blood flow. Sludging can significantly increase your risk of having a heart attack.

How might being Type A, angry, and nonmindful while eating a high-fat meal bring on a heart attack? When you're angry, your system thinks you're being physically threatened. To prepare you for a fight, circulating fat isn't metabolized in the liver; instead, it's diverted from your digestive system and gets shunted to your muscles. As a result, more fat circulates in your bloodstream. At the same time, to stop the bleeding your body is expecting from the fight, norephinephrine, a chemical messenger, increases, causing platelets to get stickier. With more circulating fat and stickier platelets, there's an increased chance of a blood clot and thus an ensuing heart attack.

What is still more telling about this study is that the more easygoing and more mindful Type B's had a more healthful response to consuming a high-fat meal: they weren't as likely to experience sludging. This fact suggests that, in general, if you happen to consume high-fat foods but you do so in a calm, relaxed, present frame of mind, you're less likely to clog your vessels, and your risk of heart disease will be lower. It would be tempting to interpret the above to mean that consuming high-fat foods won't clog your arteries if you're calm, but heart disease is multifactoral, and research is too premature for us to make this leap.

From Facts to Flavors

Such studies suggest that what you chew on mentally when you eat may be just as important as what you literally chew on. Therefore, spicing food with focused, mindful attention as you eat might make room for what in Hebrew is called *Yetzirah*, the spiritual awareness of unity and connection. In this way, food and mindfulness release their healing potential. Slowing down long enough to experience the subtleties of food is an ageless tradition. In the West, many of us limit our focus on food to its numbers (such as calories) and nutrients (fat, protein, and so on). But not all cultures share the same perspective; instead, many have a "mindfulness meal heritage."

I realized this while listening to a lecture at the First International Conference on Tibetan Medicine, given in 1998 in Washington, D.C. What I heard reframed my focus on food and mindfulness in yet another way. During a presentation about Tibetan medicine and food, an American participant who appeared to be a proponent of raw, uncooked foods, asked Tibetan physician Dr. Namgyal Qusar a question about the "ideal" diet: "Are you saying that even when food is cooked and eaten hot, there are still sufficient nutrients?" she asked. "This isn't our concept," responded Dr. Qusar. "When [Tibetans] talk about 'balanced,' we say you have to eat all kinds of food: vegetables, cereals, fruits, meat, and milk products, but we also mean at the same time that you have to eat all six tastes; otherwise you'll be missing nutrients." Dr. Qusar continued by clarifying the six tastes: sweet, sour, salty, bitter, pungent, and astringent.

What a 180-degree turnaround from Western culture's eating-by-number consciousness. Rather than analyzing food quantitatively for its nutritional content, in essence, Dr. Qusar was saying that Tibetan nutrition uses a finely honed sense of taste to ascertain whether a meal is balanced. What a wonderful, instinctively mindful and sensual way to view complete nutrition! Within the framework of the Tibetan nutrition system, eating optimally includes consuming foods from various food groups but also focusing your attention on the flavors in the food as you eat them. This mindfulness of taste has permeated Eastern cultures for centuries. Not only is it integral to Tibetan medicine, but focusing attention inside your mouth while chewing — so that you experience all six flavors — is a nutrition concept that's also integral to Chinese cuisine, traditional Chinese medicine, as well as India's Ayurveda (the "science of life") medicine system.

As a matter of fact, the six tastes are so integral to Ayurveda, that even the order in which you consume the six tastes is important. "Some ancient Ayurvedic schools maintain that the sequence of tastes in a meal should progress in the order of sweet, salty, sour, pungent, bitter, and astringent," writes Ayurvedic practitioner Maya Tiwari in *A Life of Balance*. "More recent Ayurvedic thinking, however, supports a sequence similar to that followed in the West: begin with salty and sour, progress to pungent followed by bitter and astringent, and end with sweet," writes Tiwari.

Savoring the Six Tastes

Not too long after I learned about identifying the six tastes, I had a chance to put the concept into practice. While eating at our favorite local Thai restaurant, Larry and I ordered a unique appetizer salad called Miang Kam, but what arrived at our table were not the familiar mixed vegetables. Instead, the elegant waitress presented us with a platter of small bowls, each filled with a sampling of delicately chopped, colorful food: lime, peanuts, red onions, red pepper, ginger, and roasted coconut. Fresh spinach leaves rested nearby, while in yet another bowl was some thick, sticky, sweet-and-sour paste. We were delighted with the presentation but didn't know how to proceed. Our hostess kindly demonstrated for us. As she did, eating mindfully took on an even deeper dimension. Taking a single spinach leaf in the palm of her hand, she first spread a thin layer of the paste onto the leaf. Carefully and intently, she sprinkled a tiny portion of each food over the sticky paste. Then she rolled up the spinach leaf, creating a small food-filled tube. After repeating the ritual, she laid one of the tubes on my plate, then placed the second on Larry's plate.

When we tasted the handmade "tubular salad," our taste buds were bursting with flavor. The sensation was similar to watching a spectacular, colorful fireworks display. But instead of an explosion of colors, each bite released a distinctive implosion of flavors. During the next half hour, Larry and I continued to create our own Fourth of July flavor-filled spinach roll celebration. With each creation, both our attention to and anticipation of the fantastic flavors and tantalizing tastes kept us focused and attentive throughout our dining adventure.

Stages of Success

What are the steps to eating mindfully, with conscious, intentional awareness, the antidotes to judgment, impatience, and task-stacking? Three distinct stages are necessary for moving into mindfulness — and staying there: intentionality, or deciding to be mindful; commitment, pledging to stay mindful; and focusing, remaining aware of and being in the moment.

ᐧᕵ *Intentionality*. The first step to creating mindful meals is deciding to focus on food and eating and on their connection with your social, emotional, spiritual, and social well-being. By simply becoming aware that you intend to do this, you're taking the first step toward becoming more mindful.

ᐧᕵ *Commitment.* Once you decide to be mindful, if you find your attention wandering or you are becoming distracted by judgment, impatience, or task-stacking, gently let go of the thoughts or actions that are interfering with your intention and commitment. Then remind yourself that you're committed to remaining mindful and in the moment.

ᐧᕵ *Focusing.* Holding your intention and commitment to mindfulness, focus your attention on the food or food-related activity. To further enhance your focus, use one or more of your senses: look at the food, its colors, its placement on the plate; listen to the water boil; smell the aroma of the spices; touch the utensils. All the while, remain aware that you're remaining aware by focusing.

It can be difficult to implement these three stages, because once you intend to create a meditatively mindful meal, the mind tends to become occupied with ideas, plans for the future, reflections on the past, or other thoughts or particular feelings. Remaining in the present or being mindful can often be more challenging than many of us suppose. In fact, being mindful can be so difficult that it's really a lifetime practice.

It is possible to reap the rewards, though, through the process itself. The key to success is keeping in mind that once you have the intention and your thoughts begin to crowd out the silence you're seeking, gently remind yourself of your commitment to the moment. Then focus on each moment of the meal: planning, preparation, eating, digestion, and cleaning up. Eliminating the pitfalls of judg-ment, impatience, and task-stacking calls for a major switch in think-ing about yourself, others, and food itself. You'll find, though — as I did — that replacing judgment and impatience with mindfulness is well worth the effort.

Nonjudgment in Action

Once while I was working on mindfulness with a client, she told me how she made the "leap into mindfulness" each time she ate by applying the three "stages of success." She derived this eating style of mindfulness by following her intuitive sixth sense to access the all-encompassing gratification that mindfulness can bring. Formerly filled with food-related judgment (what she should and shouldn't eat, feeling guilty when overeating, worrying about weight), with a longtime habit of working at her computer during both lunch and dinner, she learned to successfully use intention, commitment, and focus to transform an automatic-pilot approach to food into a satisfying adventure of mindfulness.

When we talked more about this accomplishment, she told me about an experience she had while listening to a consciousness-raising meditation tape as she ate a snack. Perhaps seven or eight min-utes into being enveloped by the soothing voice on the recording, she was feeling calm, relaxed, and peaceful, definitely "mindful of the moment." Then, suddenly, to underscore how judgment can affect emotional well-being and peace of mind, the moderator changed direction: "Think of a situation or person who recently upset you."

"My peace of mind ended abruptly. I left the meditation tape and began to focus my attention on how angry I was with a friend," the woman said.

"Then what happened?"

As she reflected on the question, her brow furrowed, "I was no longer feeling fine and meditating on the moment," she said. "Instead, I got emotionally lost in an upsetting situation that had happened weeks ago. And as I thought about my insensitive friend, I no longer felt peaceful; instead, my anger flared up."

"Did the meditation tape leave you in this state of mind?"

"No. It brought me back to feeling peaceful and attuned to the moment. But I still couldn't stop thinking about what my friend *should* have done in this particular situation."

"And afterward, what happened?"

"I realized that when I thought about a stressful situation, I wasn't enjoying my food. I also grasped that I wasn't really hungry. Actually, I fathomed that when I ate filled with judgment and anger, the food didn't seem to digest easily. For the first time, I realized that my angry, judgmental state of mind actually caused me to lose my appetite, that my body wasn't welcoming the food."

Before gaining these insights, my client had always thought that eating mindfully meant following behavior modification principles: turning off the TV, chewing thoroughly, setting the fork down between bites, looking at the food itself, or focusing on how full she was or wasn't feeling. Surely, these are aspects of mindful eating. But they're not the whole picture. When she was able to discern that judgmental thinking "didn't feel good," she decided to try to remain relaxed while eating (intention), to let go of negative feelings should they arise (commitment), and to stop other activities while eating (focus).

Most people who eat mindfully and enjoy their food do the same: they trust and follow their own finer instincts and inner cues to decide what works for them. As judgment falls by the wayside and they learn simply to be with and to savor each bite, anxieties and concerns about food are replaced with pleasurable peace of mind...and the promise of health.

Creating Meals Mindfully

Every time you eat you have an opportunity to take a reflective pause and to turn each aspect of your meal into a stream of non-judgmental moments of mindfulness. The more sincere your intention, and the more committed you are to participating in being present in the moment, the greater is the likelihood that you'll create meals of mindfulness. To reap the rewards, remember that creating meals mindfully is a process. Although it's not likely that you can remain mindful every moment of every meal, a great deal of awareness is within your grasp. The following exercises provide start-up suggestions for consciously and intentionally eating mindfully.

❧ *Brew some tea.* If ongoing mindfulness seems daunting, start with small, familiar steps. (Hint: your senses can help.) To begin, make a cup of your favorite tea — perhaps herbal, green, or black. Steep it for two to five minutes while waiting and watching patiently. When the tea has been brewed, savor its scent by inhaling deeply. Then notice the color: Is it green, dark brown, or almost black? Sip the tea, enjoy it, and focus on the flavor, the warmth, and the comfort it brings. What sounds do you hear as you swallow? Meditate on the moment of swallowing: How does your throat know when and how to perform this incredible feat that we take for granted? Is the tea hot or warm? What kind of aftertaste does it leave? As you sip your tea, consider saying a silent *gatha* — a simple, short phrase used by Buddhists to help focus the mind. A well-known *gatha* for drinking tea is: "A cup of tea in these two hands, mindfully held upright. Body and mind are in the here and now."

❧ *Visualize the meal.* Mentally focus on all the steps involved in making a special meal for friends or family members: planning the menu (perhaps Italian, Mexican, or American fare?), shopping for ingredients (at the supermarket or local farmers' market?), prepping the food (chopping, mixing, thawing), cooking (such as baking, grilling, broiling), setting the table (will you have a theme table, such as autumn?), serving (what steps are involved to ensure the food will be ready at the right time?), and cleaning up afterward. When will you prepare the meal? For how many people will you be cooking? Will you make something low fat and light, such as a mixed green salad? Or, instead, are you opting for a high-fat, calorie-laden quiche? Or is today the day to try that new vegetarian chili dish you've had on your to-do list?

Once you decide on what you're going to prepare, in your mind's eye, focus on its appearance (such as color), aroma, flavor(s), texture (crunchy, chewy), and so forth. If other thoughts enter your mind, such as, This will take too much time to prepare, simply witness the thought until it passes, then bring yourself back to visualizing the meal.

🐾 *Prepare food with awareness.* Often the actions we perform while cooking become automatic. Preparing meals mindfully means you're taking your actions off automatic pilot by breaking them into little steps, then consciously and intentionally observing each thought and action. For example, as you think about preparing a summer salad, focus your intention on gathering the ingredients by silently repeating the name of each vegetable: mixed greens, carrot, mushroom, red pepper, radish, cucumber, avocado. As you select each vegetable to chop into bite-size pieces, focus on opening the refrigerator, then repeat silently, "turning, opening the door, looking for the vegetables, reaching for the carrots..." Throughout the preparation of the salad, notice and acknowledge each intentional step while silently stating each action involved. Some examples: mixing salad, flavoring vegetables with dressing, placing vegetables on the salad plate, putting plates on table. Notice how long you can keep your attention focused on the food and what distracts you.

🐾 *Practice an "eating meditation."* Using the ordinary experience of eating a raisin, meditation expert Jon Kabat-Zinn takes people at his stress management clinic on a journey of self-discovery about mindfulness meditation by teaching them how to cultivate attentiveness while eating. The following sense-filled exercise is a composite of his classic eating meditation.

To begin, place a single raisin in the palm of your hand. Look at it carefully as if you've never seen a raisin before. Inspect it closely and from all sides, smelling the raisin deeply, touching it with your fingertips. Feel your body's reactions, such as salivation from merely anticipating that the raisin is going to be eaten. Then place the raisin in your mouth. At the same time, feel and sense the movement of your arm muscles that guide your hand in getting the raisin to your lips. Taste the rich and subtle flavors that the soft raisin exudes as you begin to bite into it, while noticing the role that breath plays in the taste. As you chew, notice how your tongue and the walls of the mouth are helping. Beginning to swallow, notice the delicate movement of the throat muscles as the raisin gently slides down toward its destination in the stomach. Sense the lingering aftertaste in your mouth. Throughout the process, listen to what the raisin sounds like through all its changes.

❧ *Clean up carefully.* Vietnamese Zen master Thich Nhat Hanh says, "I know that if I hurry... the time of washing dishes will be unpleasant and not worth living. That would be a pity, for each minute, each second of life is a miracle. The dishes themselves and the fact that I am here washing them are miracles!" From clearing to cleaning dishes, regard the dishes, your motions, and each action of the entire process. To help you do this, repeat the following *gatha* as you clean up: "Washing dishes is like bathing a Baby Buddha, the profane is sacred. Everyday mind is Buddha mind."

Recipes for Mindfulness

At its core, the mindfulness message is exquisitely simple: when you plan a meal, plan a meal; when you chop vegetables, chop vegetables; when you wash dishes, wash dishes; and when you intend to eat mindfully, eat mindfully. As the following stories suggest, recipes for mindfulness can be used almost anytime, anywhere.

❧ *Pouring water.* When I was in college, a friend of mine who was a teacher at a local Montessori school invited me to visit her in the classroom. Curious about how one would go about teaching toddlers, I gladly accepted. When I arrived, my friend told me that she was about to begin the water-pouring exercise that was on the day's curriculum.

As the lesson began, I watched, transfixed. With concentrated attention, toddlers and little children struggled to master the skill of pouring water from a small, plastic pitcher into a small plastic glass. Before they were allowed to try this hands-on exercise, my friend first demonstrated and discussed the procedure in a way that would make sense to a small child: look at the pitcher and the water in it; look at the empty glass; hold the glass in one hand; grasp the handle of the pitcher with the other hand; lift the pitcher; move the pitcher closer to the glass; place the spout of the pitcher against the top rim of the glass; hold the glass tightly; slowly begin to tilt the pitcher; keeping the spout of the pitcher against the glass, continue pouring until all of the water in the pitcher is in the glass; place the glass with the water in it on the table; put the empty pitcher down next to the glass.

As expected, most of the children managed to spill either a little or a lot of water as they attempted to master this new technique. Over the years, I would reflect on the exercise as I realized — more and more — that on the surface, the lesson was about teaching children how to pour water from a pitcher into a glass. But, with an adult's hindsight, I realized that practicing how to pour water held a more intangible, multifarious reflection: water gives life to both food and human beings. When it falls haphazardly from the sky, it nourishes the earth and animates seedlings, but it takes mindfulness and focused attention for human beings to contain its fluidity and to benefit from its life-enhancing nourishment.

❧ *Making tea.* About the subtle, contemplative, poetic practice of the Way of Tea, Kakuzo Okakura has written that, "Teaism is the art of concealing beauty that you may discover it." Intrigued by such a harmonious concept, while I was writing this book, I took a ten-week course on the centuries-old practice of the Japanese Way of Tea. Offered at the Green Gulch Farm Zen Center's traditional Japanese teahouse in northern California, the course was designed for those who wish to experience the ancient practice of tea more deeply. Not surprisingly, the optimal way to experience it is through the filter of a continuous stream of mindfulness meditation.

By the time I arrived at the teahouse each week, the teacher and apprentices had cleaned the tearoom, arranged freshly picked local flowers in the *tokonoma* (alcove), and made a charcoal fire. As the water boiled, each apprentice began to learn the multitude of studied steps that go into the process of both preparing tea and serving it with a Japanese sweet. Over the weeks, I received instruction in walking meditation, sitting, being a guest at a tea gathering, preparing thick green tea *(koicha)*, serving a sweet, and sharing a bowl of tea and sweet with others in the teahouse. But there were also invisible lessons.

As the course progressed, I realized that learning the Way of Tea is a lifetime endeavor. To think that ten two-hour sessions are adequate for understanding this ancient art is comparable to believing that looking into the night sky through a telescope empowers you to know all that's possible about the stars. I also learned that the more mindfulness I brought to each movement and moment, the more often I experienced a fleeting glimpse into how the study of tea releases the aesthetic wisdom of the spirit. For the Way of Tea is not only a microcosm of the universe; rather, it is a path for penetrating the puzzle of both the outside world and the awesome wisdom within.

❧ *Pizza possibilities.* My friend David Leivick is a long-time vegetarian who is passionate about food. He often cooks for his wife, Linda, and daughter, Sarah. His specialty is pizza, which he has been making each Sunday evening for more than twenty years. David shared with me his thoughts about his pizza-making rituals and recipes as well as his attention to the details of preparing pizza — all of which evolved over the years as a natural outcome of his regard for food.

"Some of my earliest food memories are around pizza. I grew up in Washington, D.C., but because both my parents were from New York City, we'd often go there to visit family in Brooklyn. On these trips, an enormous treat for me would be a visit to the local pizzeria with my cousin Steve. We'd sit at a little Formica table and watch the guy behind the counter throwing the pizza up in the air. I must have been only seven or eight, but I felt very grown up eating pizza in a restaurant without my parents.

"After college, I started cooking more and more; eventually I learned how to bake bread. One rainy Sunday afternoon, I thought it would be fun to make a pizza. Soon it became a regular Sunday evening meal for my wife and daughter. And now it's a family tradition that has continued for more than twenty years.

"I realized early on that it's not that hard to make a pizza — but it's not that easy to make a *good* pizza — especially the crust. It's basically a lifetime process to get it right: the amount and kind of yeast you use, the type of flour, and the temperature of the oven are all crucial for success.

"When the yeast proofs and starts to multiply, it's like watching the act of creation, the 'big bang.' I love to knead the dough, knowing that I'm creating something. A kind of magic happens as the flour, water, and yeast transform into something that didn't exist before.

"Over the years, I've made all kinds of pizza, such as totally green toppings made with green zebra tomato sauce, green pepper, zucchini, and green olive. Another time I made an orange-topping pizza with golden jubilee tomatoes. To enhance the color, I added some chanterelle mushrooms and beautiful orange peppers. I've gone through phases where I thought the pizza shouldn't have any cheese on it, and so I made a vegan, plant-food only, pizza. I've made pesto pizzas and dessert pizzas with muscat grapes. I've even made pizza when we've gone camping. In the summertime, I serve the pizza with salad; in the winter, it's served with roasted vege-tables, such as brussels sprouts, carrots, little potatoes....

"When I first started making pizza, I'd buy some ready-made sauce. Then I began making the sauce from scratch, using canned tomatoes. Now in the summertime, when fresh tomatoes are available, I make sauce with fresh organic tomatoes, either from our garden or the local farmers' market. When I find an array of organic heirloom tomatoes in the market, I can them so we're able to enjoy them with pizza and other dishes all year long.

"I have no intention of achieving the perfect pizza; the pleasure is in the process of working toward it — somewhat like the platonic concept of perfection. I think everybody has their own pizza, something that they work on, something that brings them continued satisfaction over a long period of time.

"For me, cooking is amazingly pleasurable. When I'm making pizza, I'm in a state of being, rather than doing. My complete concentration is on something other than myself. There's something soul satisfying about creating a good pizza. When I'm making pizza there's no other place that I want to go. I'm not on my way home — I *am* home.

chapter five

The Healing Secret of Appreciation

Be grateful for food and its origins — from the heart.

*Because food is what it is, it is of utmost importance that we
receive it with deep gratitude, because we consume life.
Whether it's cabbages or cows, it's life that we consume....
How can we not be grateful for the life that sustains us?*

— Zen master John Daido Loori

The healing secret of appreciation, the second spiritual nutrition
secret, plants yet another invisible, spiritual nutrition seed that
grows beyond mere thought. Because this secret has brought me so
much fulfillment, not only with food but in all aspects of my life,
I'm especially eager to share it with you. As you develop a deeper
understanding of it, you too will find that the more heartfelt reverence you bring to food, the richer and more meaningful will be
your experience of food and eating.

As enthusiastic as I am to tell you about this healing secret, I'm
equally disheartened about the way in which we take gratitude for
granted. After all, the soul-satisfying healing potential of gratitude
is probably the most overlooked and ignored of all the healing
secrets of food. Don't most of us approach food matter-of-factly, taking its power to sustain us for granted? And if we do take the time
to say a blessing or prayer before eating or to express thankfulness

for the food in front of us, aren't many of us merely saying words rather than speaking from our heart?

As this chapter unfolds, I want you to begin to bring your awareness from your head to your heart. This subtle refocusing — a gentle shift from mind to heart, to caring about food and of feeling appreciation for food — is pivotal to reaping the rewards of spiritual nutrition. You can implement the other healing secrets we've discussed so far — dining with others; being aware of feelings before, during, and after eating; and practicing mindfulness, but it takes being grateful for food and its origins — from the heart — to turn eating into a transformative experience that allows your soul to soar.

In the last chapter, the focus was on bringing a heightened awareness to all food-related activities. But adopting mindfulness by itself isn't enough to reap the full benefits of the healing secrets of food, because spiritual nutrition also includes allowing the heart and mind to work together by feeling gratitude for the food of which you're being mindful.

To have gratitude for something is to tap into the source — the life spring — of your inner wisdom. It is living in relationship to something else, adding something extra, giving something back even when it's not required. It's a commitment, like love, to give from your own centered presence — intentionally and consciously. When applied to food, it will enable you to merge each moment of your meals into a continual stream of sensory and spiritual awareness, capable of healing both body and soul. Since you're giving this regard to food, and therefore to life, you can't fail to get something back in return.

A Fare of the Heart

Helen Keller said, "The best and most beautiful things in the world cannot be seen or even touched. They must be felt with the heart." Each time you approach food, you're presented with an opportunity to feel it, experience it, and appreciate it — and its life force — from the heart. The word *appreciate* has its roots in the Latin verb *appretiare*, which means "to set a price on something." To appreciate food (or anything) is to value it highly; to be fully aware of it; to be thankful. Another definition is for something to increase in value.

Each time you're filled with gratitude for food (are thankful for it), it appreciates (increases in value). Yet this isn't how most of us perceive or experience food. Instead, we have learned to measure food's worth by calculating its quantities of nutrients. But appreciate it, and you're offered an opportunity to focus instead on the qualities and value of food in your life. Food becomes much more than a measurable product, and its value appreciates beyond what is measurable. You realize that its key role is to give you life. And that is everything.

A story from the ancient Hindu tradition, told to me by my friend Nischala Devi, author of *The Healing Path of Yoga*, eloquently illustrates what it means to approach food with love-filled, heartfelt appreciation. The parable, which is based on a true story from India, suggests that an appreciative heart empowers food to open its treasures to you — to the degree that you are willing to open your heart to the silent message in your meals.

Once there was a great man, a saint, who had a devout wife. On their wedding day, after they took their vows, she asked him if there was anything he wanted her to do in their married life, something solely for him. In response, he said, "The only thing I want you to do is this: every time you serve a meal, as you put the plate in front of me, also place a small bowl of water and a needle next to it."

During the fifty years of their marriage, every time she served him a meal, she honored his request by placing a small bowl of water and a needle next to his food. But the reason for his unusual request remained a secret, for she never saw him use either the water or the needle during their years together.

Toward the end of his life, when her husband was dying, he asked her, "My dear, is there anything I've done over the years that's caused you any pain? If so, let's resolve that now before I die." When she couldn't think of anything, he asked again. "Isn't there even a small thing that's caused you even a slight disturbance in your mind? If there is, please let me know."

This time she said: "There's just one thing. On our wedding

day, you asked me to put a small bowl of water and a needle beside your plate. And in all the years that we've been married, I've never seen you use either one. And I've sometimes wondered, What's the purpose of them?"

With a slight smile on his face, he said, "I have such an incredible respect and appreciation for the food that's given to me — and for you who has cooked it with such love and devotion — I felt that if for some reason — in my carelessness — I would drop even one grain of rice onto the table, I wanted to be able to pick it up with the needle and wash it in the water, so I could eat it and not waste it."

To me, this story expresses the profound meaning that an appreciative heart infuses not only into food but also into relationships and all aspects of life. As experienced by the husband in the story, when we approach food appreciatively and with loving intention, we go beyond mindfulness and we regard the sacred connection between food, nature, and humankind.

Thanks Giving

Over the centuries, heartfelt blessings, prayers, or simple moments of quiet contemplation have become humankind's ritualized ways of expressing gratitude for the life-sustaining nourishment that food provides. These expressions of gratitude evolved as thanks not only for the measurable and visible but even more for the invisible, immeasurable, alchemical, life-giving and life-containing mystery inherent in food.

It's easy to imagine our spiritual ancestors for thousands of years offering both passionate and compassionate deeply felt prayers of thankfulness for food, holding awe in their hearts for food and the elements on which they depended, which then — much more than now — were considered with awe. This stance is understandable, considering their great vulnerability to nature. After all, their very life hung in the balance of the elements and depended on the gift of an abundant, successful hunt or harvest. When their wishes and prayers for sustenance were granted, they likely perceived and honored it as grace, as Divine love and protection bestowed on them, as a gift from God.

I especially thought about such long-forgotten depths of appreciation as I worked on this section around the Thanksgiving holidays — when millions of Americans gather together to share a "meal of thanks" with family and friends. As we consume the lavish meal of turkey and dressing, mashed potatoes, cranberries, and pumpkin pie, few of us manage to remember from the history books that we're celebrating what began as a high-spirited harvest festival in 1621, when about fifty settlers at the Plymouth Plantation gathered to celebrate a measly but much-appreciated crop of corn, barley, and peas. Because the previous winter had been especially harrowing, the pilgrims brought a deep-felt appreciation to the humble harvest they had finally received from God that year. To share their joy, they invited almost one hundred neighboring Native Americans to their harvest celebration. After all, these were friends who had helped them through hard times.

Honoring Origins

Such deeply felt thanksgiving for food and all other gifts bestowed by the Creator of the universe is at the core of the sacred ways of Native American nations. With the intention of enhancing life-sustaining forces and eliminating life-diminishing forces, harvest rituals begin and end with prayers of thankfulness for all plant- and animal-based foods and other elements of nature. In this way, forces such as scarcity and drought are believed to be diminished and replaced with abundant crops and other gifts of nature. The following excerpt from the "Prayer for the Wild Things" by Marcellus Bear Heart Williams reflects Native Americans' heartfelt appreciation for all living things. With prayers such as this, the Iroquois expressed appreciation for both animals and plants and for the nourishment that they provide. Within the framework of this cosmology, Native Americans are not only thankful for food, but they're also grateful for the origins of, and forces that create, food: the Creator, or Great Spirit, and the spirit forces of wind, thunder, lake, sun, moon, and stars.

Oh, Great Spirit, we come to you with
love and gratitude for all living things . . .
Fill our hearts with tolerance,
appreciation, and respect for all living
things so that we all might live together
in harmony and peace.

When prayers or words of thankfulness are said with authentic regard, they serve as a medium that evokes the best of what is in the human heart. Vietnamese Buddhist monk and teacher Thich Nhat Hanh expresses such intention in a Zen blessing meant to be said before eating:

In this plate of food,
I see the entire universe
supporting my existence.

When I reflect on this blessing, food becomes a gateway that opens to reveal an interconnected world, a mesh of relationships among human beings, plants, and animals, among the elements such as light, water, and air — indeed, the entire universe. To express such interpenetrating connectedness, Hanh uses the term *interbeing.* When words of appreciation for food are expressed with an authentic, heartfelt sense of all-pervasive unity (after all, both food and we human beings are life-giving and life-containing, and both food and we are mutually dependent on elements such as sunlight, water, air, and earth to survive), they empower you to begin accessing the spiritual dimensions of nourishment.

A Passionate Perspective

What makes appreciating our inter-beingness with food so powerful isn't just the food on which we're focusing but also and especially the degree to which we experience the core elements of appreciation: the *passion* and *compassion* that underlie authentic gratitude. In other words, when you penetrate the essence of appreciation, what emerges is *caring* about food. To care in such a way is inherently other oriented, because instead of focusing on your own food-related concerns, you are paying attention to the food before you by regarding the mystery of life that it contains and provides. In other words, to have heartfelt gratefulness for food and its origins calls for eating *from* the heart rather than choosing foods solely because they're good *for* your heart (or waistline, or mood, and so on). And passion and compassion are the emotions that enable you to pass through the gate of gratitude.

What is it like to care passionately about the life inherent in food, to delight in the mere thought of food, to experience food from a place of such spiritual awakening and connection that your enthusiasm for food seems boundless? K'vod Wieder, associate director of Chochmat HaLev, Center for Jewish Meditation in Berkeley, California, tells a wonderful story about *Hitlahavut* (literally "flaming"), Judaism's deep, caring passion and appreciation for not only food but for all gifts from God. It's a story that's referred to in the literature of Hasidism, an orthodox tradition originating with Jewish mystics in Poland in the mid-1700s. In the story, the highly emotional Reb (Rabbi) Levi Yitzhak of Berditchev is a guest at the Sabbath (from the Hebrew word *Shabbat*, meaning "rest") celebration of the highly respected, esteemed Hassidic rabbi Reb Baruch of Medzhibozh. The more contained Reb Baruch is the very opposite of the emotional Reb Yitzhak, who during the meal is overcome with enthusiastic passion for the food. Explains Wieder:

> Realizing that the meat and fish [served for dinner] are expressions of the Divine, the passionate Rabbi Yitzhak ...becomes entranced by the choice. At first, quietly and contemplatively, he considers his choice: the meat or the fish. Then, becoming so overwhelmed with the experience of the Divine expression through food, and profoundly moved by these two totally different creations of God, he leaps up shouting, "MEAT OR FISH, MEAT OR FISH."
>
> In his enthusiasm, he knocks the platter out of the servant's hand. And the whole platter of meat and fish flies up into the air, landing on the host's *Talit* [prayer shawl]. The guests are mortified, and look to Reb Baruch, anticipating the worst.

There is complete silence before the Hassidic Rabbi says: "I want you to know that I'm never going to wash this *Talit* again, because it has been stained by one who is flaming with passion for the Divine. May we all merit such passion, such connection."

This story highlights the spiritual food wisdom practiced by both rabbis: Reb Yitzhak realizes and regards the divinity in food and in everything, and Reb Baruch knows, deep within his soul, that heartfelt, passionate appreciation leads us closer to the mystical connection inherent in both food and God. As is evident by Reb Yitzhak's behavior during dinner, feeling such enthusiastic passion for food — from the heart — goes beyond words that you might say in a blessing; it is experiencing this connection in your being and living with the flaming passion of *Hitlahavut*. Such moments of intense affection and enthusiasm for food emerge when you put food, or somebody or something else, before yourself.

Compassionate Consciousness

If bringing the strength of passionate appreciation for food empowers you to be grateful for food and its origins — from the heart — then having compassion in your heart for both plant- and animal-based food is a parallel path that leads you to another dimension of spiritual nutrition.

To have compassion for someone or something is to feel deeply for, and to share in, another's situation or difficulties. When you bring compassionate regard to food, you're opening your heart and feeling compassion for the entire food chain, the chain of Being in nature where all life is dependent on other life for survival. You're also feeling compassion for the plants and animals that will no longer be able to grow and thrive so that you might live and be nourished.

Compassion, as an integral part of the human condition, has been a feature of mythology for thousands of years. Buddhist priest and author Joan Halifax writes in *The Fruitful Darkness* that when

Bodhisattva Avalokiteshvara, the Buddha of Infinite Compassion, saw the immense amount of suffering and ignorance in the world, he cried tears of compassion. "One of these tears was transformed into...Tara, the embodiment of...compassion in Tibet." Known as the Great Mother in mythology, the image of Tara spread through China, Southeast Asia, and Japan and became merged with local deities and other wise beings. This union produced the deities of compassion Kuan-yin in China, Kuan Seum in Korea, and Kanzeon in Japan. Their unifying thread is with compassion in their hearts; they are always "listening to the sound of the world."

Many religions espouse "listening to the sound of the world" with a compassionate ear. Consider Judaism, which defines prayer as the work of the heart, the sacrifice of the heart. In Judaism, expressing thanks is more than mere words; it's a key component of the Talmud, a collection of ancient rabbinical writings that encourages orthodox Jews to say one hundred blessings a day. The purpose of these blessings is to pay homage to, and express reverence for, the presence of God in everything — including food.

"The Jewish path is often called the Blessing Path," write authors Sara Shendelman and Dr. Avram Davis in *Traditions: The Complete Book of Prayers, Rituals, and Blessings for Every Jewish Home.* But living in a blessed state of mind, by itself, isn't the point. "While expressing blessings," continue the authors, "we must be connected to that person or object, and...in a state of...compassionate connection." To illustrate such depth of compassion, Rabbi Harold Schulweis, writing in *Rabbis and Vegetarianism,* tells a story about a new *shochet,* the person responsible for taking the life of food animals. In this story, one man asks the other why he is unhappy with the new *shochet:*

"What's the matter? Didn't he recite the prayers?"

"He did."

"Didn't he sharpen the knife?"

"He did."

"Didn't he moisten the blade?"

"He did."

"What was wrong then?"

"Well," the man said, "our old *shochet* used to moisten the blade with his tears."

Such a story illustrates God's message: if you take the life of an animal for food, do so with care and compassion for the life you're taking. Since I've been studying ancient wisdom about appreciation for food, I now feel the same degree of gratitude, passion, and compassion for plant-based food (fruits, vegetables, grains, legumes, nuts, and seeds) as I do for animal-based foods (dairy, fish, poultry, meat). After all, both contain the life force and healing properties, and both give their life — and life force — so that I can not only be nourished but also continue to live.

An "Other" Perspective

The fact that heartfelt appreciation has been so integral to our relationship to food and all aspects of life for thousands of years (as we've seen with Hinduism, Native American belief systems, and Judaism, for instance) isn't incidental — some social scientists think that focusing on food and caring about something other than yourself may be one of the most important determinants of health. Published in *Psychosomatic Medicine,* the groundbreaking research that linked being self-involved to an inability to appreciate an "other" perspective and to poor health status was conducted by my husband, Larry Scherwitz, and colleagues.

While listening to hundreds of taped Type A interviews (see chapter 4 for more about Type A Behavior) with men who had heart disease and others who were healthy, Larry counted the number of self-references: *I, me, my,* and *mine.* He used the term *self-involvement,* a word that entered the English lexicon in the 1840s, to describe the intensive focus on self, and *self-referencing* to describe the excessive use of these pronouns. The results that surfaced highlighted the health threat of being overly self-absorbed. When he compared the number of self-references with those who got heart disease, those who used first-person pronouns most often not only had more heart disease–linked chest pain but they were also more likely to actually die from a heart attack. Saying the words *I, me, my,* and *mine* isn't of itself dangerous, but people who tend to use them more frequently possess an underlying self-involvement that is often linked to hostility and thus an increased threat of heart disease. After all, when you're angry or hostile, your thoughts are often filled with what someone did to you or with viewing someone as your enemy. Such a world-view translates into ongoing self-involvement.

Here's how the "me focus" can harm over time. Ongoing self-involvement is often linked with emotions such as anger, greed, depression, and anxiety. When you live in such a high-pitched, stressed-out state, more adrenaline flows through your bloodstream. In turn, blood vessels constrict and blood pressure increases. Over time, such stress can damage your arteries as well as your heart muscle. But become other-oriented, and replace negative feelings with positive feelings of appreciation. After all, it's impossible to be filled with both gratitude and painful emotions at the same time. Instead of adrenaline, positive emotions, such as appreciation, release endorphins. Not only do these chemical messengers boost your immune system (enabling you to more effectively resist disease), they also dilate and relax your blood vessels and heart muscle.

"Each time you eat, you're in a prime position to stop viewing the world through self-focused glasses and to focus on each aspect of the food and meal instead of on yourself," says Larry. When you do, you're capturing the moment by having a direct experience of the food, your surroundings, people, and your feelings, as you're eating. Such heartfelt interconnection among yourself, food, nature, and others not only makes every aspect of life more satisfying, it may also make you potentially less prone to heart disease.

Heart Power

After decades of intense investigation, researchers at the Institute of HeartMath, a think tank in Boulder Creek, California, concur with the multidimensional healing potential of an appreciative, loving heart. Writing in their book, *The HeartMath Solution*, HeartMath founder Doc Childre and executive consultant Howard Martin state: "[Our research] has shown that when *heart intelligence* (a term describing the concept that the heart is an intelligent system with the ability to balance our emotional and mental systems) is engaged [with positive emotions], it can lower blood pressure, improve nervous system and hormonal balance, and facilitate brain function."

HeartMath researchers also claim that heart-focused techniques they've developed can lower stress hormones, raise levels of the "antiaging" hormone DHEA, and improve heart rate. HeartMath researchers point to another powerful dynamic: when your heart is filled with loving appreciation, those feelings affect your body's electromagnetic field, causing it to extend three or more feet from the body.

What does such research suggest about your health and an appreciative consciousness? If you flavor your meals with other-oriented appreciation and spice them with passion- and compassion-filled prayers and blessings, you may enhance your health and well-being each time you eat. The message is clear: tap into your innate healing "heart power" at not only mealtime, but any time, and you're choosing health over heart disease.

Attitudes of Gratitude

When busy, award-winning author Brenda Knight took the time to visit her mother during the Christmas holidays to share much-valued conversation while enjoying her mother's homemade meals, she articulated her appreciation for the time and talk spent over food with the thought "attitudes of gratitude"; later, it was to become the title of a book.

Whether planning a meal, shopping for food, preparing a particular dish, savoring the scent and flavor of a favorite food, or enjoying a homemade meal with your mom, you can supplement each aspect of your meal with a caring, compassionate, and passionate attitude of gratitude. When you do, not only will you infuse both you and your food with a deeper spiritual experience, but the healing, magical mystery of gratefulness will work through you, in you — and for you. The following paths to appreciation can show you how to go about fostering a grateful attitude.

🐾 *Say a blessing.* At its core, appreciating food means caring about it, honoring it, and seeing it as the life-giving, life-containing nourishment it is. Whenever you're around food — especially just before eating, bless the meal with appreciative, heartfelt words.

Opportunities to bless food are endless. Whether you begin the day with a glass of orange juice, cup of coffee, or cereal; eat lasagna warmed by a microwave oven at work; snack on an apple or apple strudel; shop for pre-prepared pasta after work; or eat light fare of simple, steamed vegetables for dinner, each time you're around food you have the opportunity to appreciate it. To begin, let go of worries, thoughts, plans, and so on. Then, inhaling deeply and exhaling slowly as you replace any mental activity with the pure feeling of heartfelt regard for your food, say a blessing. Choose one from this chapter or make up your own simple blessing, such as "Bless this food before me and all those who made it possible for me to have this meal."

🐾 *"Shoot" an "arrow" prayer.* Because of time constraints, more and more Americans are eating fast food — often in their cars between chores or appointments. If you find yourself crunching some nachos while driving, munching a muffin between appointments, or eating ice cream in the mall, keep in mind that consciously and intentionally appreciating food doesn't have to take too much time. If you must eat quickly because of time constraints, consider "shooting" a prayer of gratitude "at" your food with the simple Native American Senaca greeting, "Thank you for being." If arrow prayers become too common, commit to taking more time to focus on your food during future meals.

🐾 *Appreciate aesthetics.* When you appreciate the beauty of food, you're experiencing its aesthetic dimension. As in viewing a painting, seeing beauty calls for appreciating its presence with a sense of your own relationship to it. Try using your senses — mindfully — to access aesthetic appreciation:

- taste the rich collection of flavors in your favorite Chinese food dish
- see the presentation of the food on the plate: the coarse texture of the rice; the rich, red color of the tomato; the lovely pattern of the herbs on the plate

- smell the enticing aromas that emanate from freshly baked bread
- listen to the sounds of dining: the clatter of plates, of water being poured, of the hum of others chatting around you while eating in your favorite restaurant
- feel the crisp crackers in your hands and how crunchy they are in your mouth

❧ *Think appreciative thoughts.* Thought brings an intellectual level to appreciation by allowing you to place things within a particular context. For example if you knew about the personal challenges that Van Gogh experienced while painting, let's say, *The Potato Eaters* — his regard for the simple, earthy beauty of the peasant life and his love at the time for dark, somber colors — you would be able to bring a cognitive appreciation to the painting each time you viewed it. In the same spirit, when you're aware of where food originates, the particulars of how it's grown, or the effort that went into its preparation — such as the time it took for you, your spouse, or a friend to put a meal together, or the years of training and apprenticeship on the part of the chef — such thoughts can help you to further appreciate food.

❧ *Infuse meaning into meals.* In chapter 3, we discussed being in touch with your emotions before, during, and after eating. These may include memory-related feelings that could inspire you to infuse your meals with heartfelt appreciation. For instance, you may sometimes feel nostalgic about the peanut butter and jelly sandwich that your mother used to make for your school lunch; passionate about family feasts that included festive foods, such as the candied yams and homemade pumpkin pie served during Thanksgiving; or compassion for an especially busy friend who — knowing you had a particularly difficult day — put in lots of time making your favorite "comfort" dish of macaroni and cheese.

❧ *Be other oriented.* While most of us are familiar with the ritual of blessing food or offering prayers of thanks before eating, what is less apparent is that bringing a sense of thankfulness to food — from the heart — begins with putting your self-focused thoughts and feelings on hold for a while. Here are some other-oriented food strategies:

- Reflect on the care and effort that go into getting fruits, vegetables, grains, baked goods, legumes, nuts and seeds, dairy foods, fish, chicken, and so forth to your table. From the people who grow, harvest, and raise food, to those who sell ingredients, and others who plan meals, shop for food, and cook and serve it both at home and in restaurants — feel a passionate enthusiasm for the food and the human effort needed to get it to your table.
- Before eating, regard the origins of food and all the elements that make food possible: the soil in which grapes grow, the sun that shines in wheat fields, the water and rain that penetrate the roots of fig trees, the air on which both food — and we — depend. Meditate appreciatively on these elements and the mystery that enables them to infuse life into food.
- Gratefully acknowledge those who harvested the fruit, vegetables, grains, legumes, and nuts and seeds as well as those who handled the meat, fowl, fish, and dairy. Thank the farmers, farmworkers, ranchers, truckers, and grocers.
- Show gratitude to the cook who prepared your food so tastefully (including yourself, if you're the cook!).
- Relish the vivid colors of your favorite fruit and the way in which the fruit is served on your plate.
- In the produce section of the supermarket or at the farmers' market, allow the freshness, quality, and abundance of the fruits and vegetables to bring a smile to your heart. With heartfelt appreciation, gaze at the straight, green asparagus; the round, purple cabbage; the green, yellow, and red apples; the sticklike orange carrots.
- As you eat, value the vitamins (such as A, the B's, and C,) and minerals (such as calcium, magnesium, zinc) in the food that you know will nourish you. Be grateful for the discoveries about nutrition that have revealed the influence the nutrients have on your health.

❧ *Picture a perfect-meal moment.* A particular form of meditative practice (called cataphatic meditation) entails holding a specific image, idea, or word in your mind's eye, then allowing relevant emotions to center in the heart. The same meditation concept can apply to appreciating food. Imagine a perfect meal moment, a specific food-related activity when you sensed that all was right with the world. You may have felt this deep sense of well-being during the last holiday dinner with your family, when you snacked on your favorite chocolate chip cookie, while sharing the first slice of your wedding cake with your spouse, after dipping your bread into the fresh "green" flavor of virgin cold-pressed olive oil from Tuscany, or while catching up with a good friend over some soup and salad during lunch.

Or there might have been a moment when you felt touched by someone's situation, whatever it was, and during the meal you opened your heart to him or her completely. At that moment, you experienced another person's perspective, another soul, like you never have before. As you reflect on such moments, bring the feelings about the memory from your head into your heart.

Recipes for Appreciation

The key to the healing secret of appreciation lies in experiencing heartfelt regard for the great web of life inherent in food and the act of eating. For when you eat, the life intrinsic in plants or animals is a gift given to you so that you may sustain your own life. Bring such an attitude of gratitude to food, and your heart may heal — both literally and metaphorically. Here are some insights into creating appreciation recipes.

☙ *Kneading bread.* Perhaps more than any other food, simple basic bread has been linked with gratitude over the centuries. Indeed, rites of appreciation have evolved over millennia to honor the "staff of life" that has sustained both the body and soul of humankind:

- The liturgy of taking the bread and wine of the Eucharist — a word that comes from the Greek *eucharistos,* meaning "to give thanks" — is the essence of the Christian faith.
- When the Israelites wandered in the desert, they were fed

by falling manna from the sky. Today, devout Jews still recite a blessing of appreciation on the Sabbath for the gift of bread: "Blessed art Thou, O Lord our God, Creator of the Universe, Who brings forth bread from the earth."

- In Turkey, devout Muslims place pieces of leftover bread on walls, because it is considered sacrilegious for bread (and food) to be left on the ground, where it may be stepped on. To step on bread is to step on a gift from Allah.

Appreciating bread isn't only for the ascetic or religious. When I was in graduate school, a friend gave me a copy of the classic *Tassajara Bread Book* (now in its twenty-fifth printing!) by Ed Espe Brown. A pioneer of the natural foods movement in America, Brown also motivated a generation of Americans to begin baking. Since the publication of the *Tassajara Bread Book,* he has been a master chef, an ordained Zen priest, a Zen teacher, the cofounder of the gourmet vegetarian restaurant *Greens* in San Francisco, and the author of many other cookbooks.

As I scanned the pages of the *Tassajara Bread Book,* I delighted not only in the text about baking bread but also in Brown's quirky, much-appreciated, step-by-step illustrations. Inspired by the book and the author's regard for baking bread, I kept our home in freshly baked bread for almost ten years. I recently took advantage of a chance to attend a cooking class that Brown taught for an evening in a town not too far from where I lived. Although the meal he prepared was quite varied, it was his demonstration of kneading dough that transfixed me.

Perhaps the terms *bread meister* or *dough artisan* would most accurately express what I witnessed as I watched Brown knead the dough. Watching him mixing, pressing, turning, massaging, molding, and manipulating the dough was comparable to observing a sculptor create a work of art. Brown displayed confidence and ease of motion; gentle but firm regard for the dough; gentility when gathering it toward himself; firmness — but up to a point — when pushing it away; and ... always ... rapt regard for what he was doing. Ed Brown once commented during a presentation: "What is in your heart is your true nature. Let your experience into your heart and let your heart respond." The way Brown kneaded and handled the dough spoke of an intimacy with it, of a profound, symbiotic relationship he had developed with the dough over many years of bread making. Surely he had let the experience of making dough touch his heart.

Ultimately, Brown's cooking demonstration revealed more than a technique for kneading dough to release its optimal flavor and texture. He gave me a recipe for how to appreciate and regard making bread: along with flour and water, knead in some quality care, attention, and nurturing. In this way, not only do you touch the food, but you're allowing it to touch your heart.

🎋 *Wilderness wanderings.* Right from the start, the trip was a challenge. Toward the end of August, Larry and I took a three-week backpacking trip into the Weminuche Wilderness in the San Juan Mountains of southwestern Colorado. Our plan was to follow the Continental Divide trail, located twenty miles from the nearest road; ultimately, we would reach an altitude that averaged 12,000 feet. The other challenging aspect of the trip was figuring out the food we would take with us. We knew that altitude and exercise initially suppress appetite, but the high caloric demands of climbing, especially in a cold climate, would increase our desire for food.

Our staples were dried fruits such as apricots, peaches, figs, dates, apples, and pears; our favorite nuts — walnuts and almonds, pre-ground (so they would cook more quickly); whole grains (especially oats and brown rice); a colorful medley of ground legumes; and a potpourri of dried vegetables that included tomatoes, carrots, peppers, and corn. We would supplement our protein intake with powdered milk, and some soy protein (a coarse meal-like mixture called textured vegetable protein). Our snacks were granola, granola bars, and some dark, chewy chocolate.

As the trip progressed, we realized we hadn't brought enough seasonings or an adequate variety of food; nor had we taken enough to eat for a three-week trip. Because of these limitations, we both developed a deep-seated hunger and craved varied food textures, protein, rich flavors, and so on. Because of this experience, we were developing a deep appreciation in our hearts for the varied flavors, tastes, and textures inherent in food ... qualities that we had often taken for granted when all sorts of food had been readily available in our everyday lives.

We also wanted fresh food — but this was a challenge about which we were prepared to do something. Just before leaving, a friend had taught us how to forage in the forest for leafy greens and wild onions; we even found fresh, wild strawberries (they're about a third smaller than traditional strawberries). The strategy for foraging fresh food was simple: we'd seek out a flat area not far from where water flowed. Receiving fresh food from the earth opened our hearts to feeling a deep reverence for the cycle of life.

Toward the end of the trip — I think we began to hike out of the wilderness on the seventeenth day — we spent an entire day planning the food that we would take on our next trip. But, quickly, we turned to more immediate gratification and began to rhapsodize about the food we would eat when we got into Durango, a nearby, charming Western storefront town with a main street, a train depot for the Durango and Silverton narrow gauge railroad (built in 1882), lovely art galleries and artisan shops ... and exceptional restaurants.

After leaving the wilderness and arriving in Durango, right after checking into our hotel, we went straight to The Warm Flow restaurant on the main street. It was exactly what we needed at the moment: a welcoming place with wholesome food and friendly service. As we sat comfortably at a booth, we scanned the menu. Our order? The "kitchen sink," a dish that was filled with the fresh food we craved. When it arrived, our eyes fixed on a large, round platter that contained a high (translation: huge) mound of mixed, fresh vegetables (greens, tomatoes, cucumbers, carrots, sprouts, peppers, mushrooms, avocados, and so on), a sprinkling of sunflower seeds, and finely grated cheese. The "kitchen sink" also came with two (albeit small) still-warm-from-the-oven, freshly baked loaves of whole grain bread, served with organic butter. Given our sense of food deprivation in the wilderness, we felt particularly passionate about the food before us. We savored each bite, the miracle of food, the luxury of being waited on, the cozy atmosphere ...

When we finished, we ordered yet another entrée: warm, flavor-rich, baked eggplant parmesan. At that point, the waitress said, "You won't be able to eat all this." Larry's response: "We've been in the wilderness for nineteen days. Please bring it, and we'll decide if it's too much after it's served." We ate it all. Warm, baked food never tasted so good. Savoring the afterglow of the meal, we began to giggle as we both realized that the only thing that would heal our bone-deep hunger would be a sundae at the local ice cream shop. After sharing three scoops of ice cream, replete with chocolate sauce, sliced banana, whipped cream, and nuts — and topped with the requisite cherry — we finally felt satisfied.

The combination of deep hunger, a strong appetite, and calorie (and probably nutrient) deprivation had created a deep craving for fresh, nutritious, varied, satisfying — and fun — food. What a relief it was to know that we no longer needed to talk about flavorful food at night in the darkness of the tent; we could experience, sense, enjoy, and savor it "for real." Even till this day, I don't think we've ever appreciated food in such a primal, profound way.

chapter six

The Healing Secret of Connection

Create union with the Divine by flavoring food with love.

A chickpea leaps almost
over the rim of the pot
where it's being boiled.

"Why are you doing this to me?"

The cook knocks him down with the ladle.

"Don't you try to jump out.
You think I'm torturing you.
I'm giving you flavor,
so you can mix with spices and rice
and be the lovely vitality of a human being.

Remember when you drank rain in the garden?
That was for this."

Grace first, sexual pleasure.
Then a boiling new life begins,
and the Friend has something good to eat.

Eventually the chickpea
will say to the cook,

     "Boil me some more.
Hit me with the skimming spoon.
I can't do this by myself.

I'm like an elephant that dreams of gardens
back in Hindustan
and doesn't pay attention
to his driver. You're my cook, my driver,
my way into existence.

I love your cooking."

— Jelaluddin Rumi, thirteenth-century Sufi mystic and poet,
The Illuminated Rumi, *translated by Coleman Barks*

The third spiritual nutrient is the healing secret of connection, which is perhaps the most exciting of the healing secrets. Once I understood this secret at its deepest level, it changed my perception about food forever. You will discover — as I did — that embracing it not only transforms your relationship to food but to life itself. This is because applying this concept each time you eat will enrich and nourish your soul in essential, profound, and fundamental ways you likely never before expected, experienced, or even imagined. At the end of this chapter you'll learn ways to bring the secret of connection into your life every time you prepare, cook, or eat food, and you'll see how loving connection makes a difference not only to the food itself but also to your health and well-being. But for now, just ponder the idea that flavoring food with love makes a difference.

The concept of creating connection with food should be familiar to you by now. After all, throughout this book we've been discussing the connection between food and your social well-being, between food and your feelings, and between food and your spiritual sensibilities via the two other spiritual healing secrets of mindfulness and appreciation. This healing secret, however, differs from all the others we've discussed in that when you connect with food by creating union with the Divine — the mystery that is life — by flavoring food with love, your entire relationship to food takes a 180-degree turn. Instead of turning to food for what it can do for your social, psychological, and physical well-being, the core nutrition concept now becomes, What can you do to enhance the food itself and imbue it with the spiritual nutrients of love and connection to life and the cosmos?

Flavoring Food with Love

I first became aware of the significance of connection when I had the privilege of talking with Hindu cardiologist Dr. K. L. Chopra, father and mentor of well-known author Deepak Chopra. At the time, I was in New Delhi, India, where I had been invited to give a nutrition workshop at the First International Conference on Lifestyle and Health. During our discussion about Hinduism and food, Dr. Chopra commented: "*Prana* is the vital life force of the universe...and it goes into you, into me, with food. When you cook with love, you transfer the love into the food and it is metabolized [when you eat]." Dr. Chopra based his beliefs on the Bhagavad Gita, the Hindu scripture that encourages cooking food with love. I found it amazing that Hinduism, a 3,500-year-old religion, tells us that a loving consciousness affects food, and not only this but also that we might "metabolize" this loving energy — our own, or someone else's — each time we eat what I call "spiritually imbued food."

By now I'm sure you realize that the term *spiritually imbued food* doesn't apply to traditional vitamins and minerals; rather, I'm talking about the nutrients that may manifest when your heart is open, when your intention is focused, and when you are fully experiencing loving regard during the preparation or consumption of a meal. This concept also applies to having loving regard for all those involved in food preparation — from farmers and grocers, to home and restaurant cooks — as well as to those who eventually eat the food. We have myriad opportunities to impart a spiritual consciousness (loving awareness and intention) into our food.

Connection Clues

We need only to look in our own backyards to discover the truth about this spiritual nutrition concept. Clues that consciousness does indeed influence our food are all around us. As a matter of fact, such a seemingly mystical union between consciousness and food may be more common than we suspect. For example, it has filtered into our culture via literature. Remember author Laura

Esquivel's charming novel (and movie) *Like Water for Chocolate,* a mystical melodrama about the effect feelings have on food and on those who eat the food? Throughout this story about the passions of young love, those who eat meals prepared by the heroine seem to be overcome by the very same feelings she had while cooking the food. (Who can forget the scene of the wedding guest filled with sadness after having eaten wedding cake "flavored" with the tears of the groom's true love?) Or consider the movie *Chocolat,* a charming fable about the power of chocolate to instill loving feelings even into those who are seemingly most resistant to its love-laced magic.

Another, more personal clue that preparing or eating food with loving regard makes a difference surfaced years ago when my husband and I first began to use our new food processor. Independent of each other, we both came to realize that the food (carrots and mushrooms, especially) we touched and prepped by hand — with attention and care — had a fuller, richer flavor than the processor-chopped vegetables; somehow, the vegetables that we prepared by hand also created a more soul-satisfying eating experience.

But the message that food could be spiritually imbued was really brought home to me years later when Larry and I attended a workshop in Hawaii led by Leonard Laskow, M.D. Based on the concepts described in his book, *Healing with Love,* the seminar was designed to teach course participants how to heal both self and others with a technique Dr. Laskow created that uses subtle (loving) energy in our bodies to heal. One day during the workshop, Dr. Laskow showed us how to apply his healing-with-love method to wine; on another day, we repeated the experiment with an orange. To begin, he held his hands close to the food or liquid, taking care not to actually touch it. He visualized a golden ball of light above his head; then he drew this "golden energy" through his head, into his heart, and then into his hands.

During the next few minutes — keeping his hands close to the wine flask — he thanked the grapes for "allowing" themselves to be made into wine; he also thanked and acknowledged all elements (such as the soil for its nourishment and the sun for its energy) and people involved (from the grower to the trucker) in bringing the wine to us. Throughout this procedure, he continued to envision the golden energy being infused into the wine. Then Dr. Laskow set the wine aside for about ten minutes, as you might do when you marinate some food, so it could "reconstruct." After the wine or orange was infused with loving, golden light, participants had a chance to taste the "treated" wine and orange and also some that were untreated. We could all detect distinct differences in the scent, flavor, and body of both the wine and the orange. To me, the spiritually imbued wine and orange smelled and tasted subtler and more gentle, not unlike a lovingly prepared dish that had been made with quality ingredients.

In essence, by having the intention to impart loving energy into a food or beverage — and then visualizing this happening — we seemed to have brought about a noticeable change. Not only did the spiritually imbued wine and orange taste different from the untreated items, but I seemed to have metabolized this loving energy. For after imbibing the loved-infused wine and orange, I also *felt* different, filled with a palpable feeling of positive energy. In short, I witnessed and experienced what appeared to be the channeling of conscious, loving energy into food.

Of course, my response may have been due to my expectations that the treated wine or orange would taste better. In other words, the change could be attributed to the expectancy effect: I *expect* the flavor of the wine or orange to change after it's been infused, so it does. Even so, we all had the same experience: the taste, fragrance, and texture of the treated wine and orange were different. Interestingly, when I repeated this as a double-blind experiment with students at a course I taught at California Pacific Medical Center's Institute for Health and Healing in San Francisco — in which nobody knew which wine was "love infused" — every participant detected a difference in taste and scent in the infused wine.

A Double Dose of Love

Even though I've repeated this experiment successfully many times during my own workshops, I am still awed by the incredible concept that we may transmute loving, conscious energy into food and beverages as well as ingest this energy when we eat. Is it really possible — as Dr. Chopra suggested — that some form of energy within our systems can be transferred to our food, changing its form by adding a thought or feeling, a different subtle quality or vibration? If so, the implication is that not only does food affect our bodies but also that we influence food, too, making eating a two-way communication.

Here's how this "double dose" of communication works. When you bring a loving regard to food (or to virtually any relationship in your life), first you bless yourself with the loving energy before you direct it toward the food. In turn, the food or beverage receives this energy; then when you eat this love-flavored food, you are again nourished in some special way (which we'll discuss later in the chapter).

In terms of the concept of connection, the three elements that we are uniting, or with which we are interconnecting, are a loving consciousness, food, and the Divine (however we may perceive of it: the life force, the Absolute, the Supreme Being, the Creator, the Higher Self, God, the mystery that is life itself, and so on). When you imbue food with the invisible substance of love, you're mingling with the real, authentic, underlying value and meaning of food. When you recognize food as a life-giving, life-containing manifestation of the mystery and beauty around us, you're realizing and honoring your "sameness" and "oneness" with it. In essence, this is what it means to practice the healing secret of connection: creating union with the Divine by flavoring food with love.

The Eating-Papers Story

Others have experienced the mystical healing secret of connection in unusual ways. For instance, Larry Dossey, M.D., executive editor of *Alternative Therapies* medical journal, tapped into it via a love-infused tablet he ingested after he'd been hit by a severe health-robbing bug. I think you'll find his experience as intriguing as I did.

In 1992, while presenting at a health conference in Baja California, Dossey became severely ill. Far away from home, he suddenly felt feverish, faint, and so weak that he had trouble standing or walking. Making his way back to his room, he collapsed on the bed. The illness continued to progress, and he soon became wracked with bone-shaking chills and a high fever. As a physician, he suspected that some toxin or pathogenic organism had attacked his blood or tissues. But instead of turning to traditional emergency medical care for treatment, he did something that was both faith filled and brave: he asked a trusted friend, whom he considered to be a "born shaman," to treat him by writing some healing (confidential) words onto a small piece of paper. The "born shaman" was Frank Lawlis, a member of the *Alternative Therapies* advisory board.

Without reading the words, Dossey then asked his friend to fold the paper tightly into a size comparable to a tablet. Chasing the "tablet" with a glass of water, he swallowed it as he would any other medication. Then, feeling well cared for, he lay back and drifted into unconsciousness. During the next three days and nights — semidelirious, too weak to talk, and feeling he might die — Dossey drifted in and out of consciousness. Along with the singular paper tablet, the only addition to his dietary regimen was the consumption of fluids. And then he began to recover, although it would take weeks after his return home for him to feel normal again. It was during this time that he learned that he had not gotten as ill as the others at the conference who had been afflicted with the same symptoms.

"In choosing to ingest words scribbled on paper, I had not dreamed up a new therapy," writes Dossey in *Alternative Therapies*. "I was invoking an ancient healing custom...that reflects history — the eating of prayers, Bible verse, or magic formulas.... The slips of paper are called *Esszettel* ('eating-papers') or *Essbilder* ('eating-pictures' or 'eating-images')." Dossey concluded: "The eating-papers might have served as a vehicle or intermediary device for the empathic intentions, thoughts, wishes, or prayers of the person administering them."

Dossey's experience may be interpreted several ways. First, there is the possibility that he may have gotten well even without taking the tablet. Also, his belief and expectation that the love-infused paper tablet could help heal him might actually have promoted healing —

the placebo response. Another interpretation is that the intentional healing energy infused into the paper by Dossey's shaman friend and colleague actually had a direct healing effect once the tablet was consumed.

Regardless of the interpretation, each points to the same possibility: that directing intentional energy (in this case, wishes for healing to take place) into nourishment (whether it's food or a paper tablet) may have an effect on health and well-being. Whether you're consuming a paper tablet, food, or a beverage that's been infused with love, the implication is the same: it seems possible that we do, indeed, metabolize the loving regard with which they've been imbued.

Plants Feel?

As unique as Dr. Dossey's experience is, the idea that our consciousness, in some mysterious way, influences food — or even paper — is more mainstream than many might realize. For instance, do you recall, in the 1970s, when we were told that if we talked lovingly to our plants they would grow better? Some of us giggled as we admitted to friends that we were, indeed, watering our plants while talking to them lovingly. Feeling somewhat ridiculous, some of us continued to forge ahead anyway. And if our houseplants thrived, we began to believe that we had found the secret to having a green thumb.

The idea of talking to our plants penetrated the culture when polygraph examiner Cleve Backster showed that plants actually do seem to respond to our feelings. Backster's adventure began through a fortuitous set of circumstances in the 1960s, when he impulsively attached electrodes from his polygraph to the leaf of a dracaena plant, a tropical plant with large palmlike leaves. When he watered the leaves, the galvanometer registered a reaction. Amazed by the idea that plants might react to how they were treated, he tried a few more experiments. He formed an intention in his mind to burn the leaf — and imagined the flame — and the polygraph needle jumped. He had not lit a match or even moved a muscle.

Since Backster reported his amazing finding that plants can

detect our intention, he has continued, and other researchers have followed suit, performing dozens of experiments on plants and food. Indeed, the research discussed in the classic book *The Secret Life of Plants* by Peter Tompkins and Christopher Bird confirms that some kind of instantaneous communication between human beings and plants seems to exist, suggesting that plants and other forms of food may indeed "read" intentionally directed mental energy.

For instance, another example of this dynamic occurred when Backster cracked open a raw egg that he planned to feed his Doberman. While opening the egg, he noticed a "strenuous reaction" from one of his plants attached to a polygraph. When Backster observed the same reaction the next evening, he attached an egg to a galvanometer. For nine hours afterward, the chart continued to record an active response from the egg. The conclusion? "He appeared to have tapped into some sort of force field (between the egg and the plant) not conventionally understood within the present body of scientific knowledge," write Tompkins and Bird.

Water Works

If plants and food somehow sense and respond to verbal and nonverbal communication from humans, is positive, loving communication with plants the secret to having a green thumb? Research by Bernard Grad suggests that it is. While working at a psychiatric institute in Montreal, Grad conducted a unique experiment to ascertain the effects of feelings on plant growth. He had a clinically depressed patient and someone with a green thumb each hold a flask of water in their hands. Then he watered plant seedlings with three different samples of water: one held by the depressed patient, one held by the green-thumb patient, and the third sample of plain, untreated water.

The seedlings watered with the "green-thumb" water grew fastest, those with the "depressed" water slowest, and those with plain water somewhere in between. Many experiments later, "Grad saw the implications of his experiment to be far-reaching," write Tompkins and Bird. "If a person's mood could influence a... solution held in the hands, it seemed natural to assume that a cook's...mood could influence the quality of food prepared for a meal."

Because the human body is about two-thirds water and most edible food has a high water content, the implications for this research are quite significant. For instance, if water is changed in some way by our emotions — as Grad's studies suggest — then might not our state of mind influence both the water-filled cells in our body as well as the food we eat?

Of Prana, Chi, and Dharma

What exceptional power are we witnessing here? Hindus use the Sanskrit word *prana* to describe consciousness and the invisible life force; in Chinese, *chi* is the word that reflects the divine energy of life in all things. Devout Buddhists describe this essence of life as dharma (the teachings of Buddha, universal truth, the balanced way of nature). As applied to food, Abbot John Daido Loori, an ordained priest and teacher, says: "At the very moment of eating, we merge with ultimate reality. Thus dharma is eating, and eating is dharma."

Kakuzo Okakura has described *chi* as something that began "at the great beginning of the no-beginning." It is the same mysterious life energy and force that allows us to create union with the Divine each time we eat. In its conception of *chi*, Taoism encourages us to approach food with loving intention so that we may move beyond the level of thought and sense the sacred connection among Mother Earth, food, and humankind. "When you appreciate food from this place of spirit, your heart is open, and the chemistry of the body, I imagine, burns food in a different way," psychologist and Tao practitioner Michael Mayer speculated. Cultivating *prana, chi,* or *dharma* is both an art and a science, giving us the capability of releasing insights, intuition, and a sense of unity among mind and body, self and food. Although you may not have described it with these words, many of us have experienced this profound sense of oneness and connection that can occur. This feeling of oneness can happen anytime and anywhere when you are open and attuned to the experience of eating (or any other mystery that is part of life).

For instance, I often experience this sense of unity when I hear profoundly beautiful music that touches my heart and soul. Although I don't understand Italian, as I listen to Italian tenor Andrea Bocelli sing certain arias (or anything at all on his *Romanza* album), I feel a sense of oneness with life. I listen mindfully to the music, appreciating — from the heart — the beautiful song and Bocelli's extraordinary voice. And then, perhaps for only thirty seconds or a minute, a certain succession of notes and words somehow speak to some truth within me. When this occurs, I am completely in the moment, lost in the soaring message that seems to reside both within and between each note. Time stops, and all that remains is the beauty of the music and the invisible, universal message, the connection between the music and me. At moments such as these, I am filled with a sense of well-being, love, and spiritual connection with the world. Am I in touch with — moved by — *chi, prana,* dharma, the Divine or Absolute, the mystery of life? Absolutely.

Maybe you're asking, What do such lofty spiritual concepts have to do with food? Nurse Joyce Zerwekh defines spirituality as "the essence of personhood, the longing for meaning in existence, the experience of God and of ultimate values. Its ultimate end is union or connection with a reality more enduring than the individual self." Zerwekh's definition of spirituality suggests that by transcending the self, we access the mysterious energy of life. In the last chapter, we discussed the powerful heart-healthy implications of transcending the self by becoming other involved, by regarding food with both passion and compassion. When we do, love itself becomes an expression of self-transcendence. In turn, we transmute both food and ourselves, and in the process, create a deep and fundamental connection to the food we eat.

Yoga-Flavored Food

As amazing as the results of all the research are, the truth is that our spiritual ancestors have turned to food as a medium between loving consciousness and the Divine for millennia.

Consider the yogic philosophy of the sage Patanjali, who codified *The Yoga Sutras,* a classic, concise compass of the main practices of yoga (meaning "yoke" or "unite"). To lead practitioners to spiritual union with the Divine, the yoga philosophy suggests various paths, including knowledge (*jnana* yoga), work (*karma* yoga), physical poses, or asanas (*hatha* yoga), love (*bhakiti* yoga), and meditation (*raja* yoga). But yoga encompasses much more than paths for achieving union. Huston Smith, author of *The Illustrated World's Religions,* describes the connecting, infinite, subtle energy pursued by yogis and other mystics very poetically: "I am smaller than the minutest atom, likewise greater than the greatest. I am the whole, the diversified-multicolored-lovely-strange universe. I am the Ancient One, the Lord. I am the Being-of-Gold. I am the very state of divine beatitude."

Both yogis and Hindus believe that each time we eat we have an opportunity to access "the Ancient One." Hindus see the world as a hierarchy of interpenetrating substances that enable ingested food to become a potent medium for transmitting these substances. Viewed from this spiritual vantage point, eating is transformed into a sacred act — one that is both an expression of love and a connection to the soul. Hindus and yogis alike share a profound appreciation for the interaction between food and a vast web of invisible interconnected threads. They believe that everything we eat or drink has a vibrational quality to it — as does the person who cooks the food. Because of this, when devout Hindus or yogis prepare or cook food, they do so with a loving consciousness. This means, conversely, that if your thoughts are disturbed by anger, fear, or other negative emotions, it's best not to cook or eat until you're in a better frame of mind. Why? Yogis believe the vibration of the cook's feelings goes into the food.

Some yogis even suggest that we should refuse to eat food that was prepared by someone in a negative state of mind. When we spoke, former swami and international yoga master Nischala Devi offered this advice: "If you hear a cook arguing in the kitchen, that's the best time to get up and walk out of the restaurant, because he or she is putting that negative vibration into the food just as surely as if they were dropping poison in it."

In my workshops, I've discovered that many people are amazed by these ideas. But once we do our own hands-on, double-blind experiment with wine (each person samples "love-infused" wine and untreated wine, unaware of which is which) and course participants taste and smell the change in flavor and fragrance for themselves, they often recall their own experiences with spiritually imbued food — even when — perhaps especially when — the food has been flavored with negativity.

For instance, once when I was giving a three-day workshop on the ideas discussed in this book, one of the participants shared a cooking experience that demonstrated the potent power emotions may have on the outcome of a favorite food. "You know, Deborah, your state of mind really does make a difference when you cook," one course participant told me. I listened with interest.

"Every Christmas I bake fresh cinnamon rolls for my family," she continued. "I cook them with care, and really do spice them with love. They're so good, they've become a delicious family tradition that my children and husband look forward to. But this past year, for the first time, the batch of cinnamon rolls didn't come out well. Actually, this is an understatement; they were terrible. The yeast didn't seem to have much of an impact; not only didn't the rolls rise when I baked them, they were also hard and tasteless. Because nobody ate them, I threw them out."

As we continued to talk, I asked her why she thought this happened. "I now remember that when I was mixing the ingredients, my husband came into the kitchen, feeling super angry about something. And so I put the baking on hold while we had a fight, a big fight," she acknowledged.

I considered her experience, reflecting for a brief moment on my own cooking fiascoes that may have been caused by negative energy while cooking. However, while listening to her story, I also considered more practical explanations: that the failed cinnamon rolls were caused by yeast that wasn't produced at the right temperature or perhaps because of other mechanisms about which neither of us were aware. Still, the possibility remained: Had the cinnamon rolls been ruined because they had been spiced with negativity?

"Were you able to make reparations to your disappointed family?" I asked.

"Absolutely," she responded with a big grin. Wanting to keep up the family tradition, she made another batch the next morning after her husband and she had made up.

"And they were delicious?" I asked expectantly.

"They were as good as ever, even better," she said. "And they disappeared quickly."

Meal of Mystery

Let me tell you about another kind of meal, one that has been soul satisfying for millions of people. It's a "meal of mystery" that has been prepared with love for thousands of years. I am referring to the Christian tradition of the Eucharist: infusing bread and wine with love as a means of merging with the Divine. This ritual, as many of you know, has been at the core of Christianity since the Last Supper.

What exactly is the mystical aspect of this ritual, which has captured the imagination of Christians for thousands of years? Catholics describe its mystery as transubstantiation, changing the Eucharistic bread and wine into the body and blood of Jesus Christ. When Catholics participate in the taking of the Eucharist, they approach the holy table with love in their hearts for God and Jesus. While ingesting the wine and bread, they're "taking in" the spiritual sustenance of Jesus' godliness and presence. By ingesting the body (bread) and blood (wine) of Christ, Catholics believe that the love of God is entering directly into the cells of their bodies. Protestants, however, interpret the word of God itself as direct communication with human beings. Whether you view transubstantiation as symbolic or as a profoundly literal Divine union, the underlying truth is the same: food serves as a medium that unites our loving consciousness with Divine love.

Echoing spiritual sentiments similar to that of Hindus — and alluding to *chi, prana,* and dharma — nun Hildegard of Bingen wrote about the consecration of wine and bread in the twelfth century: "We cannot see that secret vital force...which gives life to the grape and the grain." Yet "the same force is at work when the bread and wine of the Eucharist are transformed into the flesh and the blood of Christ."

Some people have been so momentously moved by the taking of the bread and wine of the Eucharist that the experience irrevocably changes them and, ultimately, their lives. When she was a child, Jean Molesky-Poz, a practicing Catholic and former member of a Franciscan religious community, experienced just such a connection. Currently a lecturer in ethnic studies at the University of California, Berkeley, she told me about her first encounter with the Eucharist at age seven: "I was at a church in San Bruno, California, and had not yet taken my first Communion. But during a eucharistic service, I actually remember feeling this overwhelming presence of being loved, and that I would be held in that kind of love forever. I recall being taken into another time and place at that moment, of being filled with love. Something in my soul had been touched." Carrying this memory and loving awareness into adulthood, Molesky-Poz later joined the Franciscan religious community.

Indigenous Insights

The concept of connection and interrelationship between our consciousness and food has permeated virtually every culture. Nowhere is this reverential connection perhaps so all-encompassing than for native peoples. This includes northern and southern Native American Indians and members of indigenous tribes such as Australian aborigines and Pacific Islanders. For tens of thousands of years (compared to the major wisdom traditions, which are less than five thousand years old), these peoples have experienced and understood such a total interconnection and union between themselves, other sentient beings, the elements (such as wind), and all of nature that they regard the universe as one "family."

Termed *wakan* by Sioux Native Americans and described as *everywhen* by Australian aborigines, this sense of primal spirituality and interrelationship of course extends to animals and plants, which are also perceived as family. Senacas, for instance, believe that all crops were given to them by their Creator *(Hawenniyuh)*. So integral to family is corn, that eastern Indians of North America perceive the spirit of maize as a woman, sacred texts of the Cherokee sometimes evoke corn as "the Old Woman," and the Huichol Indians of Mexico imagine maize as a little girl.

Because for native people plants and animals are family members with spirits, when a tribal hunter pursues food, the act goes way beyond seeking satiety. In a similar attitude of reverence as that held by Jewish and Muslim believers, native hunters turn the hunt — from the concept itself to the way in which the animal is slain and consumed — into a ritual of meditative prayer and appreciation for both the process itself as well as for the life given by the animal. In essence, native peoples perceive the earth and the web of life as sacred and both plants and animals as interconnected parts of the universal whole. Writes Smith: "The primal world is a single cosmos that sustains its embryos like a living womb."

The "I-Thou" Food Friendship

In his famous book *I and Thou,* Jewish professor and philosopher Martin Buber put into words a landmark philosophy about a spiritual connection that has been a part of Jewish beliefs about food for thousands of years. In essence, Buber's philosophy (which evolved from Hasidism) addresses the way in which we experience life in relation to God, nature, and other human beings. And this relationship is determined by our consciousness — meaning the thoughts, feelings, and awareness with which we relate to living entities.

Though Buber's philosophy mainly concerns human relationships, it also applies to an attitude toward life as a whole, and thus we can extend the analogy to our relationship with food. For instance, if you see food as an object separate from yourself, as just "fuel" to be analyzed and ingested, Buber might describe this attitude as an "I-It" relationship. But if you perceived food in relation to yourself, to nature, and to God, as something with which you meaningfully interact, Buber might call this connection an "I-Thou" relationship," or "the cradle of the Real Life."

At the heart of Judaism's dietary laws is the tradition of keeping kosher — eating certain foods prepared in a particular way. What does Buber's philosophy imply about these ancient laws? While it would be easy to dismiss them as outdated and unnecessary, they are actually an intricately worked tapestry that infuses food with meaning. A closer look reveals that they actually reflect a profound reverence and compassion for all life, that they're a "golden thread" linking the food we eat to an I-Thou awareness and compassion for all life.

Rabbi Harold Schulweis of Temple Valley Beth Shalom in Encino, California, uses the term *refined consciousness* to express the sacred sense of connection that Judaism's dietary laws ask Jews to bring to food, especially animal-based food. While the Hebrew Bible tells us that our initial diet was plant based, as civilization grew, so too did humankind's propensity for eating meat. Indeed, Rabbi Schulweis told me that before the advent of Judaism's dietary laws — in a world of animal sacrifice and ritual, hot weather, and no refrigeration — it wasn't unusual for people to consume meat without regard to the welfare of the animal's life and well-being. In response, God gave Noah and his descendants permission to be carnivorous, but because animals are creatures of God, their life (and death), the biblical dietary laws tell us, should not be taken lightly. Explains Rabbi Schulweis: "God is saying, If you must eat meat, do so with awareness that you are taking the life of another. If you must take the life of another, see to it that it is done with compassion."

What Can Food Show and Tell Us?

Gleaning wisdom from ancient cultural and religious traditions is but one way to gain insights into the healing secret of connection; tuning into the silent message in our meals is another. Do you recall being in grade school and participating in show-and-tell? Some students would show the class something special; others would tell a tale of personal interest. Scientific experimentation with plant-based food may be able to show and tell us something about the potential interconnection between food and human consciousness.

Consider the photographs of food taken by Harry Oldfield and Roger Coghill, discussed in their book *The Dark Side of the Brain*. These photographs aren't typical, familiar pictures of food; rather they're based on Kirlian photography, a special photographic technique that can capture the naturally occurring radiation field (electroluminescence) that surrounds not only food but all the cells of our bodies. According to Oldfield and Coghill, the more energy in these fields, the more potent is the life force of the cell in the biological system (such as plant or human).

When Oldfield and Coghill applied Kirlian technology to various cooking methods, the food "showed" that the (biophoton emission) field surrounding fresh, uncooked food was much brighter and larger than the field that emanated from cooked food of any kind. Their results of various cooking methods — ranking from highest to lowest natural radiation fields — is cooking with a wok, steaming, microwaving, pressure-cooking, deep-frying, grilling, and oven-baking.

I was intrigued when I mulled over these results. But at first I couldn't determine why food cooked in a wok would show more powerful energy fields than that prepared by other methods. Why would wok-prepared food seem to be more potent than steamed or pressure-cooked food? Perhaps a potentially powerful dynamic is at play. Remember, from the previous chapter, the (measurable) energy field that emanates from your heart center? With that in mind, isn't it likely that when you prepare food in a wok at close proximity, you must do so with a consciousness of careful regard and attention or the food will burn? And while you're cooking and tossing and turning food in the wok, isn't your heart center close to the food? Given these conditions, might this have something to do with how we flavor food with love, as Hindu cardiologist Dr. K. L. Chopra suggested? Might love-infused food be the secret behind the visible energy that is emitted via Kirlean photography?

I realized what food might also potentially tell us about the spiritual union of food and feelings one evening while talking with biophysicist Beverly Rubik, who had joined my husband and me for dinner in our home one evening. Dr. Rubik is the founder and president of the Institute for Frontier Science and the author of *Life at the Edge of Science*, in which she writes, "Dozens of laboratories around the world have studied a wide variety of species of plants...and have collected a substantial amount of experimental evidence that (they) emit a weak biological light."

During the course of our conversation, Dr. Rubik recounted a story that suggested that food did, indeed, communicate with us in some way. In Dr. Rubik's case, this intercommunication occurred when she was conducting research in Germany with healers who were exploring the effects of imparting healing energy to soybean sprouts. In this double-blind study, Dr. Rubik at first did not know which batch of sprouts had received healing energy. But in a darkened chamber, using a sensitive light-measuring instrument, she was able to observe that some of the sprouts (the treated ones) emitted more photons of light from the leaf tips and the root hairs than did the others (the untreated sprouts). Later, when Dr. Rubik observed a healer sending loving energy into about-to-sprout soybeans, she could both see and hear the sprouted soybeans actually snap open, emitting a just audible "clicking" sound. In other words, they appeared to respond to intentional loving energy with a click and an eagerness to grow.

Metabolic Mysteries

Just how powerful is the notion that infusing food with loving consciousness makes a difference to our health and well-being? So far in this chapter, we've discussed nutritional anthropology and scientific studies. More typically, however, in our culture the concept of loving consciousness is framed within the context of prayer and faith as powerful medicine rather than as a specific link to food. But there are similarities between these approaches. After all, as with spiritually imbued food, isn't prayer really about filling your heart and soul with love and compassion?

Praying evokes beneficial changes in the body; for instance, blood pressure, heart rate, and metabolism decrease. But not only does a loving, compassionate, prayerful consciousness influence our physical well-being directly, it also impacts bacteria, which can be found in food (as well as in our bodies). This became evident when members of Spindrift — an organization that studied prayer and its effects — went to Haiti to work with the rural poor. The lack of refrigeration meant they had trouble keeping milk fresh. Although they didn't get the refrigeration they prayed for, their prayers were answered in another, unexpected way: the milk started staying fresh for days longer.

To date, scores of studies have been done on the impact of loving consciousness on bacteria, all of which suggest that it does, indeed, affect its growth — and potentially our food and health. In fact, the faith-healing connection has so permeated our culture, that as I write this book, almost 50 percent of American medical schools offer courses on the increasingly meaningful subject of faith and healing.

What else might we infer from what ancient wisdom and state-of-the-art science have to tell us about the healing secret of connection? "Love gets around," says Larry Dossey, who has written several books about the power of prayer, consciousness, and spirituality. "Assuming a compassionate, loving attitude toward food not only has effects on the food in terms of freshness and so on, but the way your body metabolizes — whatever that is; it is a mystery." Dossey is a pioneer in an emerging field that studies the effects of prayer and consciousness on healing. Although this research is in its infancy, certainly the physical evidence consistently shows that plants can both receive and respond to intentionally directed energy emanating from humans. Indeed, scientific studies are beginning to support what believers learned intuitively ages ago: that our thoughts, feelings, and intentions seem to influence — and connect us with — the sentient, living world around us in many subtle ways; that we can enhance our lives and our food with these energies; and ultimately that it is, indeed, possible to create union with the divine when we flavor food with love.

Creating Conscious Connection

Are these concepts amazing? Absolutely — unless you've experi-enced them for yourself. It's possible for you, too, to access this energy in your heart, mind, and soul each time you eat. In chapter 8, I'll show you how to put all the healing secrets together into one, complete, step-by-step, optimal eating meal meditation. For now, it's enough for you to recognize how easy it is to create union with the Divine by flavoring food with love. The exercises and mini-experiment below are beginning steps to learning how to become a pathfinder on the road to creating conscious connection with your food.

❧ *Pursue peacefulness.* To embark on the conscious-connection journey, make it a point to let go of all negative emotions and thoughts when you're around food. For instance, when shop-ping for vegetables, preparing pizza, or eating an enticingly deli-cious dessert (such as chocolate cake or a chocolate chip cookie), do so in a calm, peaceful, and pleasant frame of mind. Simply put, for those moments when you're around food, commit to stopping all the emotional busyness in your mind and replace it with loving regard for your food.

❧ *Connect with the mystery of life.* As discussed in the chapter on food and appreciation (chapter 5), connection includes gratefulness for all that went into creating the food we eat. Before eating, acknowledge the interrelationship and connection of all liv-ing entities — including yourself — who have had contact with the food: soil (which produces plants that nourish human beings and animals), water (a key component of all edible food as well as of human beings), plant-based food (fruits, vegetables, grains, legumes, nuts and seeds), food animals (cows, fowl, fish), and food intermediaries, such as farmers, truckers, grocers, chefs, friends, and family. As you experience this interconnection, you are begin-ning to create conscious connection with your food.

❧ *Imagine food in its original form.* Visualize the food in front of you in its initial incarnation. Look at your bread, and pic-ture the golden wheat shafts blowing in the breeze; taste the potato and imagine the scent of the tubers as they're pulled from the earth; take a bite from the proverbial apple and see the sun shining on the apple tree. If you're eating animal-based food, imagine the cow grazing in the field, the fowl flying, or the schools of fish swimming upstream.

🦋 *Infuse food with love.* Whether you're eating a momentous Thanksgiving meal — trimmings and all — snacking on some celery, baking bread, or cooking couscous, hold love in your heart and loving intention in your mind. Continually flavor any food with love, regard, and appreciation that's before you: on shelves in the grocery store, in bins at your local health food store, while you're cooking a casserole, while heating up some hot chocolate, or as you're recharging after a busy week at your favorite restaurant. Regardless of the setting, remain mindful of the gift of food. Imagine that this regard is flavoring your food. Throughout your meal or snack, continue to infuse the food in front of you with loving regard.

🦋 *A mini-experiment:* As a contrast to the above connection exercises, the next time you prepare or eat a special food or dish that you've previously prepared or eaten lovingly, choose to do so — this time — during an especially busy, anxious time in your life. For instance, prepare (or eat) the dish while under pressure to meet a deadline at work. Or perhaps you're in your car, munching a snack as you rush to pick up your kids. Just be sure that the loving regard for the food is missing and instead is replaced with emotions such as anxiety, a sense of urgency, anger, frustration, disregard, and so on.

Can you detect any difference between the regarded and unregarded food? Do they taste different? Also, how did you feel — both physically and psychologically — after consuming either the "positive" or "negative" food? Did you experience a difference in the way in which the food digested or in how you felt afterward?

Recipes for Connection

My colleague Michael Mayer coined the expression "eating from a place of spirit" to describe what it means to create a conscious, loving connection to food. Ultimately, it calls for activating a sense of oneness — not only with food but with others and all else that surrounds us. Following are some recipes for creating conscious connection with food. The secret ingredient: the degree to which you are willing to be aware of your food while opening your consciousness to the love in your heart.

❧ *A taste of India.* Like an old attic brimming with collected family treasures, Indian food is a rich repository of ancient, love-filled wisdom that opens a door to the past. Yogi O. M. Aivanho reflects such sentiments: "While you eat, think of food with love, for that will make it open its treasures to you." Indeed, in India, imparting a consciousness of love to food is a major consideration for practicing yogis and devout Hindus alike. Given this belief, the person cooking the food plays an important role.

Intent on honoring India's food philosophy — one of the oldest on earth — I decided to cross the threshold from Western to Eastern cooking. I decided to invite some special friends over to share an Indian meal and to steep it in India's love-filled tradition. The occasion was especially meaningful to me, because my first book, *Feeding the Body, Nourishing the Soul,* had been inspired by a conversation I'd had with a devout Hindu about infusing food with love. Indeed, it was the subject of the entire book. While writing the book, I'd experimented with infusing food and beverages with love, so I knew that doing so did, indeed, influence both flavor and aroma. But so far my personal experiences with this technique had been limited to oranges, water, and wine. So I approached the first, full, love-infused meal I would make with unrestrained enthusiasm.

Out of respect to Indian cuisine, instead of thinking gourmet this and epicurean that, I took the opposite route. I would rely on the simple foods typical of Indian cookery, fresh ingredients that are essential to the preparation of authentic Indian food. Here is my menu:

- *Appetizer:* marinated slivers of carrots
- *Lassi:* yogurt drink, flavored with rose water and mango juice

- *Sag paneer:* creamy spinach dish made with soft cheese
- *Raita:* grated-cucumber-and-yogurt dish, flavored with chopped coriander leaves, cumin powder, and black pepper (although this is typically a cooling, refreshing side dish, I served it as a first-course soup)
- *Sadhu:* chickpea curry, cooked in lite coconut milk and spiced with ginger, turmeric, cumin, cinnamon sticks, cardamom pod, bay leaves, jalapeno chili, jaggery
- *Purusha:* brown basmati rice mixed with chopped cashews, sauteed raisins and onion, cinnamon, and ground saffron
- *Chapatis:* round bread patties, made with whole wheat pastry flour
- *Chutneys* (supplemental, powerfully flavorful accents): apple chutney, made with green apples, jaggery, and red chili and date chutney, blended with grated ginger, lemon juice, and water
- *Dessert:* homemade banana and coconut sorbet

On the surface, creating the meal was a whirl of activity: planning the menu, shopping for intriguing ingredients, and then chopping, stirring, spicing, mixing, blending, kneading, and tasting. Then I set the dining table with taupe linens, impressionistic dinnerware, and gold-plated utensils; all the while, crystal glittered from the lighted chandelier above the table. The last step to set the culinary stage: I placed sweetly scented flowers (white narcissus) on the table and more dramatic ones (deep red gladiolas) in the living room.

Meanwhile, my inner world was a complete contrast to my outward busyness. Silently, intentionally, and continually (as often as possible), I infused each phase of the meal preparation with an awareness of the union between food and us human beings; I perceived each moment as an opportunity to savor the process and the gift of life that enabled me to create the meal; with each gesture, my heart remained deeply connected to the nourishment that food provides; and always, I meditated lovingly on the food.

As the meal evolved, I realized that only by looking deeply into each detail of the meal-making process could I begin to glean the whole of its multidimensional nourishment. Then, when the meal was ready and warming in the oven, the table had been set, and I'd lit the last candle, the doorbell rang. My dinner guests had arrived. When I asked my friend Linda Gibbs to share her memories of that evening, this is what she said: "I knew we were in for a treat when my family and I stepped into your warm and inviting home and were greeted with unusual and delectable scents coming from the kitchen.

"Throughout the evening, everything was served with care, beginning with the mango drink and hors d'oeurves that we enjoyed in your living room. Also, it was apparent that everything was carefully and consciously prepared, that you had paid attention to every detail of the evening.

"The food had an earthiness and goodness about it. It was not pretentious, yet it was sophisticated in its complexity of tastes. I felt as if something different were going on — an awareness or consciousness within the food. Everything was delicious and it was one of the most memorable dinners I've had."

❧ *Office food offerings.* What do you get when you mix the three elements of spiritual nutrition (mindfulness, appreciation, and connection) with a special bring-your-own brown-bag office lunch? Answer: a soul-satisfying food odyssey — at work! Such a concept may seem like an oxymoron, but during the years when my husband, Larry Scherwitz, was the director of research at Dean Ornish's Preventive Medicine Research Institute, practicing and implementing spiritual nutrition concepts were integral to the way in which Larry and a few colleagues typically dined during the day.

The unusual office dining adventure evolved because, at the time, Larry was researching the Ornish lifestyle program, the first to show that it's possible to reverse heart disease through the lifestyle changes of a no-fat-added, plant-based diet; exercise; stress management (yoga and meditation); and social support. Over the years, some volunteers who wanted to use their internship to qualify for medical or graduate school had joined Larry's research team; part of their requisite training was to practice the components of the reversal lifestyle program. The rationale was that by learning how to practice and share this program, they would have an opportunity both to internalize and to understand it — and, ultimately, to better help patients they may treat in the future.

Because Larry was profoundly familiar with the concepts of spiritual nutrition, he added the three spiritual nutrients of mindfulness, appreciation, and connection to preparing and tasting of the office fare. Not surprisingly, over the months, a particular pattern of rituals and recipes evolved. Each day, both Larry and his team would bring in a potluck dish to share with one another during lunch. Stopping work midday, they would sit around the large, round table in Larry's office. Then, while enjoying a view of the nearby harbor and marina, each one took a turn to describe and discuss the dish they had made for the day.

Š *Office recipes.* For Larry, this often included an unusual sprout salad, a mixture of "living" sprouts. To prepare it, he would purchase a colorful potpourri of uncooked, fresh legumes and nuts at a specialty Indian grocery store. During any one week, the mixture of sprouts may have included garbanzo beans (chickpeas), adzuki beans, and mung beans, as well as three kinds of lentils, and fresh almonds. Once home, he would soak the beans overnight, then water and drain them three times a day during the next several days. When the beans and almonds were moist and chewy, and they had sprouted sufficiently (which typically took three to five days), Larry would mix them together, then toss all the ingredients with the potent flavoring of asafetida powder, an Indian spice that releases an incredible burst of flavor.

Continuing to adhere to the no-fat-added plant-based fare, the volunteers might contribute such potluck dishes as a wild rice and raisin salad, grilled vegetables, fresh vegetable salads, cooked lentil dishes, or perhaps a nutrient-dense bean brew, which might include pinto beans, chunks of acorn squash, carrots, fresh corn from the cob, and a medley of flavorful spices.

Š *Spiritual nutrition in action.* After each person had described the food and ingredients in the dish he or she had prepared, they would share insights that may have surfaced as they had prepared the dish. Here is a sampling of mindfulness-based discoveries: finding a new, unfamiliar food, tasting the food's crunchy texture for the first time, or observing how the natural sweetness in vegetables was released when they were grilled.

Expressing appreciation manifested as the group recited an ancient Sanskrit prayer of appreciation before eating: "Beloved Mother Nature, You are here on our table as our food. You are endlessly bountiful, benefactress of all. Please grant us health and strength, wisdom and dispassion to find permanent peace and joy." A side effect of the blessing was that as each person held appreciation in their hearts, he or she created connection by infusing loving regard into the food.

❧ *After-lunch "digestif":* It isn't unusual for Europeans to enjoy a digestif after dining — an herb liqueur believed to enhance digestion. In lieu of liqueur, the spiritual nutrition group invented its own after-eating digestif: Instead of immediately rushing back to work after eating, everyone sat around and talked about how much they appreciated the meal and how good they felt about creating such conscious connection with both the food and one another. In this way, Larry and his research team turned the midday meal at work into a social, soul-satisfying dining odyssey — and a lunchtime spiritual retreat...and treat.

chapter seven

The Healing Secret of Optimal Food

Eat fresh whole food in its natural state as often as possible.

Part of me wants to go back in time . . . creating a golden world of fresh food, gorgeous ingredients, wholesome food with flavor. Where people laugh and are really happy as they eat.

— Restaurant critic Patricia Wells,
"A Gourmet's Recipe for Culinary Bliss"

How ironic! The sixth healing secret, which demystifies what to eat for optimal health, isn't really a secret at all. In fact, it's a message with which we've been inundated. I still consider it a secret, though, because *we're not getting it.*

The health-enhancing healing secret of optimal food can be expressed simply: eat fresh, whole food in its natural state as often as possible. To ensure that this guideline isn't interpreted as more dietary dogma, or as more rules and regulations for you to follow, I've qualified this secret with the phrase "as often as possible." My intention is to help you think of a variety of fresh, whole food as your "most-of-the-time" way of eating, not as yet another diet to follow for a while before returning to your usual way of eating.

I'm happy to be telling you about this healing secret, because it will serve as your nutritional compass and life preserver, the guideline that will enable you to take charge of what you eat — with confidence

— regardless of the "diet du jour" or conflicting scientific insights. Keep your eyes on the signpost that reads *fresh, whole food,* and whenever seemingly contradictory nutrition information threatens to guide you down the wrong nutrition road, this easy-to-follow healing secret will keep you from getting lost in the inevitable nutri-babble.

A Return to Real Food

As you become more familiar with this secret, there's a key concept to keep in mind: you'll enhance your ability to benefit from the foods we'll be discussing in this chapter if at the same time you integrate the social, psychological, and spiritual nutritional wisdom discussed so far. Such an approach is the essence of integrative nutrition. This means that the previous chapters about the healing secrets of socializing, feelings, mindfulness, appreciation, and connection planted a nutritional crop filled with seeds about how to eat for physical health and social, emotional, and spiritual well-being; in contrast, this healing secret harvests nutritional wisdom about what to eat for physical health.

As with the other integrative nutrition insights, this healing secret is designed to further transform and broaden your relationship to food. But in lieu of more dietary numbers, what follows are general conceptual guidelines about optimal food; some insights into both ancient dietary wisdom and state-of-the-art science; and suggestions for how you may benefit by making fresh, whole food the mainstay of your diet.

Beyond being about eating integratively, the healing secret of optimal food also demystifies what has become a complicated, confusing nutrition guideline. By clarifying what optimal foods are and how they enhance health, I hope to metamorphose the dietary confusion that has reigned for so many Americans into a crystal-clear nutrition concept. You'll no longer need to depend on somebody else's diet to decide what to eat; rather, you'll be empowered to create your own optimal eating strategy. As a matter of fact, after you become familiar with the nutrition concepts in this chapter, as with the other healing secrets, you'll no longer perceive food as components of a "diet." Rather, food will return to its rightfully integrative, health-enhancing, soul-satisfying place at your table.

Which Do's and Don'ts to Follow?

My message throughout this book is that our myopic, calorie-counting approach to nutrition takes into account only one-sixth of the story. Although food and nutrition are a six-part gift, when most of us "open" this gift, we peek at only one corner. As a result, we're drowning in a profusion of one-sided nutritional knowledge, and confusion reigns about what exactly constitutes optimal food.

The sometimes contradictory smorgasbord of dietary do's and don'ts adds to our bewilderment. For instance, margarine used to be perceived as health promoting; now, because of its trans-fatty acid content, it's thought to be harmful. Further, the 30 percent fat dietary goal — eating only 30 percent fat a day to lower odds of heart disease, cancer, and other ailments — isn't only vague and arbitrary, it's become questionable. Indeed, the kind of fat we consume is considered as important as the amount of dietary fat we eat as a predictor of health and well-being. Even as I write, confusing, conflicting nutrition advice continues to permeate the media. For instance, over the decades, the high-protein, high-fat fad diet (eating mainly dairy, meat, chicken, and fried food) was replaced with a call for a low-fat or no-fat-added diet of predominantly complex carbohydrates (fruits, vegetables, whole grains, and beans and peas). But now, "carbs" and lean cuisine are again out of fashion, and the high-protein diet has again reared its unhealthful head.

Consider the cover story in a recent *Time* magazine: "Low-carb diets: meat-loving, bread-banning regimes are the rage. Do they work? Are they healthy? Here's the skinny." But the "skinny" itself is contradictory. Qualifying his support of the high-protein, high-fat diet for weight loss in the article, which was entitled "How I Became a Low-Carb Believer," author Woodson C. Merrell, M.D., writes that he still has "a hard time recommending a [high-protein], high saturated-fat diet to [his] patients. I am concerned about its effects on people with serious heart, liver or kidney disease and cancer." He continues with this warning: "As long as you're healthy, a high-fat, [high-protein] diet is usually fine for a while. But after about a month, you should go off it." Does that seem like supportive, positive advice about a high-protein, high-fat diet from a "low-carb believer" to you? It sure doesn't to me.

Confusing, conflicting nutrition advice abounds. Some other highlights: a study published in the respected *Journal of the American Medical Association* (JAMA) suggested that men who consume a higher-fat diet, which includes artery-clogging saturated fat, are less likely than men on lower-fat diets to suffer strokes. Yet another headline from a local paper tells me that "dietary cholesterol isn't bad after all," while still another declares that "the egg taboo is beginning to crack." Translation: we're now being told that cholesterol-laden eggs are okay for healthy people. Such advice appalls me, given that about 50 percent of people who have had heart attacks weren't aware they had heart disease; in other words, they thought they were "healthy."

Coping with the Conflict

With such a plethora of adverse advice surrounding us, I'm not surprised that many of us are bewildered about what to eat for optimal health. In response, frustrated Americans have taken action by deciding to eat from "both sides of their mouths." One side is consuming nonfat food products as never before: sales of nonfat Snackwell's cookies have surpassed those of America's former favorites, Oreos and Chips Ahoy. At the same time, a recent CNN report, "Food to Die For," tells us that Americans are enjoying artery-clogging desserts in droves: Ben and Jerry's chunky cookie dough ice cream is the company's bestseller; Häagen-Dazs's ice cream sales are booming.

As givens in the health and nutrition fields continue to change and controversy continues to reign, surely the solution doesn't lie in ignoring all science and, in the end, playing Russian roulette with our health. But if scrutinizing state-of-the-art research reveals that even health professionals find it difficult to agree among themselves about optimal eating, how do you find an optimal eating guideline for yourself, based on your unique food preferences, health concerns, and goals?

In other words, if our analytical, eating-by-number approach to food isn't as effective as we would like — as is evidenced by our expanding waistlines, ongoing heart disease, and the escalation of other chronic ailments such as diabetes, high blood pressure, and certain types of cancer — what then works? Is there a big picture that our nutritional myopia is keeping us from seeing? Is there long-standing nutrition advice on which the scientific community agrees, time-tested guidelines that cultural traditions, religions, and science support? Absolutely. The answer lies in three simple words: *fresh, whole foods.*

Whole Foods Demystified

What exactly are "fresh, whole foods"? Basically, they're foods that contain all the natural, original parts of the plant. Most typically, they consist of the following plant-based food groups:

Plant Food Groups	EXAMPLES
Fruits	Fresh apples, oranges, kiwis, oranges, bananas, cherries, peaches, apricots, grapes
Vegetables	Leafy greens — such as kale, chard, mustard greens — and carrots, broccoli, cabbage, and cucumber, as well as tubers (such as sweet potato)
Whole grains	The familiar whole wheat, brown rice, oats, and rye, as well as the not-so-familiar millet, barley, buckwheat, quinoa, and triticale
Legumes	Beans, such as garbanzos (chickpeas), lima beans, lentils, navy beans, kidney beans, and soy beans; and peas, such as black-eyed peas and split peas
Nuts and seeds	Walnuts, almonds, peanuts, sunflower seeds, sesame seeds, pecans, chestnuts, and filberts (hazelnuts)

Fresh, whole grains are the backbone of a whole-food diet, and many are available in both commercial supermarkets and in health food stores. Dried beans and peas, though not a typical part of the American diet, are both easily available. Depending on the season, it's easy to find an array of fresh fruit and vegetables; and nuts and seeds are most healthful when purchased in their shell.

Writing about fresh, whole foods in their classic cookbook *Laurel's Kitchen,* Laurel Robertson and Carol Flinders offer this guideline: "There are three principles [for following an optimal whole-food diet are]: variety, whole foods, and moderation. Wise choices in eating depend upon understanding [these] basic principles of good nourishment."

Of Meatlessness and Meat

Some of you may have noticed that I haven't used the word vegetarian to describe plant-based foods. This is because my intention in this chapter isn't to encourage you to become a vege-tarian; rather, it's for you to understand what foods contribute to optimal health. I make this distinction because most people become vegetarians as a commitment to ecological, ethical, and/or health concerns. Within the context of this book, the focus is health — and I've met many vegetarians who don't eat healthfully.

I realized this fact while working as the director of nutrition in Europe with my husband on what we called the European Lifestyle Heart Trial. During this time of intensive lifestyle research (based on the work of Dean Ornish, M.D.) with heart patients, I analyzed scores of vegetarian-based diet diaries. When I looked at the results, what became apparent is that it's easy to be a "junk-food" vegetarian; all it takes is avoiding animal-based foods while at the same time consuming lots of high-fat, sugar-dense, processed plant-based foods. Some examples: sugar and fat-laden candy bars, fatty potato chips, or processed grain-based foods, such as white bread and white rice. Conversely, other vegetarians may avoid added fat and sugar but still not eat enough from all the whole food groups necessary to achieve optimal health. The end result is malnourishment.

Where do meat and other animal-based foods fit into the whole-food picture? Technically, because they're not plant based, meat, poultry, fish, and dairy products aren't whole foods. If you do eat animal-based foods (which most of us do), here are three tips: 1) choose fresh animal-based foods (in lieu of mostly processed "products" such as salami, bacon, hamburger, chicken "nuggets," or fried fish); 2) begin to think of animal-based food as a "condiment" (a seasoning or flavor enhancer) rather than as the core of your diet; and 3) commit to choosing lean meat, poultry, and fish and low-fat or nonfat dairy products — as often as possible. The basic animal-based food groups are:

Animal Food Groups	EXAMPLES
Poultry	Chicken, turkey, duck, quail, pigeon, goose
Meat	Cows, lamb, pigs, goat, deer, rabbit, squirrel
Fish	Freshwater fish such as pike and catfish and saltwater fish, including salmon, sturgeon, and shellfish (clams, oysters, mussels, and so on)
Dairy	Beverages such as milk, buttermilk, and cream; and dairy products, such as ice cream, cottage cheese, hard and soft cheeses, yogurt, and eggs

Add the plant-based foods of fruits, vegetables, whole grains, legumes, and nuts and seeds to the mix, and you have all the naturally occurring food groups that exist. To achieve optimal health, the two key questions to ask yourself are:

1. Do I eat mostly plant-based foods with smaller servings of lean fish, poultry, meat and low- or nonfat dairy products?
2. Or is my eating style based on the typical American diet, that is, predominantly animal-based, with limited servings of fruits, vegetables, whole grains, legumes, nuts and seeds and high in processed, packaged foods, such as salami, potato chips, cookies, and soft drinks?

Inverse Eating

Harriet Washington writes in the *Harvard Health Letter:* "Regardless of whether [nutrition researchers] have studied the Mediterranean, China, or other parts of the world, [they] recommend that meat should be used as a seasoning and not as the centerpiece of the meal." Such a way of eating is the inverse of the American diet, which builds meals around meat, with few servings of fresh vegetables, fruits, and grains. With the typical American diet as a starting point, I use the term *inverse eating* to describe a predominantly fresh, whole, plant-based diet supplemented with small servings of fresh, lean meat, poultry, fish, or dairy foods.

Although it's the opposite of our typical eating style, outside America, inverse eating is the norm — and has been for tens of thousands of years. For instance, in spite of many Americans' perception that the mainstay of Italy's diet is white-flour pasta, wine, and buckets of olive oil, the Mediterranean diet is really another example of an inverse eating style that's based on fresh, whole foods in their natural state. The interest in the Mediterranean diet began in the 1960s, when the World Health Organization revealed that Mediterranean coastal dwellers — people living in countries such as Greece, Italy, Spain, and Portugal — not only lived longer, but, as in rural villages in China (where the diet hasn't changed much in thousands of years), they had relatively low rates of both heart disease and some cancers. Because the populace in some of these Mediterranean countries consume a high percentage of dietary fat (40 percent in Greece, for instance), these findings surprised the researchers.

To investigate the apparent discrepancy, they closely scrutinized the diet and reported the results in 1993 at a conference sponsored by the Harvard School of Public Health. The findings showed that the typical Mediterranean diet emphasizes fruits, vegetables, grains, and legumes, with low to moderate intake of dairy foods, poultry, and fish. Small portions of red meat are eaten only occasionally, and the fat in this diet comes mostly from fresh-pressed olive oil, feta cheese, and yogurt.

Asian Wisdom

Imagine beginning your day with a breakfast buffet based on *congee* — an easily digested soup that Asians have consumed for centuries — to which you add all kinds of condiments that may include pickled or salted vegetables, beans, some peas, or grated eggs. Or you might choose to add onions or peanuts. Perhaps you'll add some noodles or a small wheat dumpling to the soup. Such breakfast fare was common in classic China (before Communism). With roots in the philosophical and religious beliefs of Confucianism, Buddhism, and especially Taoism, the ancient food philosophy of China embodies all fresh food: fruits, vegetables, grains, legumes, nuts and seeds, and lesser amounts of fresh fish, poultry, and meat. At the same time, it encourages us to pursue balance, harmony, and connection with all of nature each time we eat.

My insights into this ancient, inverse culinary system were born during an intriguing conversation I had with Effie Chow, founder and president of the East West Academy of Healing Arts in San Francisco. Dr. Chow, who is a grand master of *qigong* (an ancient energy-moving healing system that is both an art and science), integrates Chinese nutrition concepts into her traditional Chinese medicine practice. "To remain balanced, we eat everything together," states Dr. Chow. "After all, this is what life is, what the universe is.

We are a tiny bit of the whole universe, so why should we just take one bit of the universe to feed only one bit of ourselves? Each cell in us represents the whole universe. And so we must partake of the whole universe each time we eat. In this way, we balance our health."

Intrigued by China's "whole-universe" diet, researchers from Cornell, Oxford, and Beijing universities spent a decade taking a closer look at the relationship between diet and health in China. Called the "China Project," the huge, long-term study began in 1983 with scientists canvassing the diets of 6,500 families in 130 rural villages. They selected this population because the villagers, who had not yet been influenced by Western food available in cities, still ate the classic Chinese diet. In 1989 to 1990, the collected data confirmed a reliance on grains such as rice (in the south) and corn, wheat, and millet (in the north); many fresh and dried mineral-dense vegetables, such as mushrooms and seaweed; and protein from soybeans and grains. With the exception of special banquets and feasts, meat and other animal foods were eaten only as condiments.

The results showed the Chinese diet to be 75 percent total calories from carbohydrates, 10 percent from protein (mostly from plant sources), and 15 percent from fat. In contrast, Americans on the average consume 45 to 50 percent total calories from carbohydrates; 15 percent from protein (most of which is from animal sources); and about 35 percent of calories from fat. What was especially surprising was the discovery that the average Chinese in rural communities consumes more calories daily than the average American. Yet obesity is very rare in China. And their average cholesterol levels are far below 160, compared to the American range of 150 to 300; and the diagnoses of heart disease and breast and colon cancers are rare.

Of course, with this study, we can't conclude that lower rates of obesity and other health problems are due solely to diet. After all, obesity could be less common because the Chinese may be more physically active, or perhaps they lead less stressful lives or have closer connections to family. Nevertheless, this study verifies that a diet consisting mostly of fresh, whole foods, with smaller servings of animal-based foods, is common worldwide and is linked to a lower risk of obesity, heart disease, and some types of cancer.

Inverse Eating and Heart Disease

The message is clear: what our bodies adapted to thousands of years ago is still optimal for us today. Perhaps nowhere is this more evident than in the groundbreaking work of Dean Ornish, M.D., and colleagues, who during the last decades of the twentieth century caught the world's attention with studies (published in the *Journal of the American Medical Association* and *The Lancet*) showing that heart disease could be reversed — without drugs or surgery — through the comprehensive lifestyle changes of a no-fat-added whole food–based diet (and stress management, exercise, and group support).

Specifically, Dr. Ornish's no-fat-added "reversal diet" consists of fresh fruits, vegetables, whole grains, legumes, and a limited amount of nonfat dairy products. Nuts and seeds aren't included, because they're too high in fat (for those who wish to help their clogged arteries). If you follow this plant-based diet — without adding any additional fat — you'll be eating 10 percent (or less) of calories from the naturally occurring fat in the whole foods.

As amazing as Dr. Ornish's research is, the program's five-year follow-up results, which were published in the *Journal of the American Medical Association* in December 1998, were even more intriguing. Research participants following the program for five years achieved an average of 3 percent reversal in arterial blockage, compared to 11 percent progression of blockage in the arteries of those following the standard 30 percent fat, American Heart Association–type diet (a lower-fat version of the typical 35 percent calories-from-fat American diet).

Worldwide Wisdom

Although various lifestyle factors (like exercise and group support) in cultures may vary, inverse eating has been the perennial dietary wisdom not only for China but for cultures and healing traditions worldwide. Here are some examples:

- The core of the Mexican diet is rice, beans, and corn, supplemented with meat, poultry, or fish.
- A typical meal in the Middle East is couscous, made with bulgur (cracked wheat) and bits and pieces of lamb.
- The core of the Japanese diet is rice and tofu (made from soybeans), which is often supplemented with fresh fish.
- People throughout India eat whole-wheat chapati bread (in India, white flour costs more than whole-grain flour), with lentils or legumes, greens, and other vegetables. Because the majority of Indians are Hindu and believe in *ahimsa* — causing no harm to animals — most are lacto-vegetarians who supplement their plant-based diet with dairy foods, especially yogurt and milk.
- Unlike America's popular version of massive, melted-cheese pie, more commonly called pizza, Italy's original version often consists of a wonderfully crusted bread, served mostly with freshly prepared, locally grown vegetables.
- When I reviewed the *Hadith,* Islam's prophetic traditions, I learned that the diet of the prophet Muhammad — the founder of Islam — was very simple: fruits, vegetables, grains (especially barley), legumes, nuts, and seeds. The milk he drank was fresh and unprocessed, as were the eggs that he ate. Because he lived simply, lamb and other meats weren't a mainstay.
- Ayurveda (the science of life) is the world's most ancient medical system, an ancient Indian healing art. With a focus on encouraging health (rather than on treating disease), its nutritional strategy takes many dietary variables into account, such as how food is prepared, food combination, the quantity of food, the season and time of day that food is eaten, and an individual's constitution (called *dosha,* defined as *Vata, Pitta,* or *Kapha,* in Sanskrit). Regardless of such personalized considerations,

one concept is constant: various, fresh, plant-based foods are encouraged for different *dosha*s; lean animal-based foods (such as turkey, fish, or egg whites) are often acceptable, while "heavy" foods such as red meat (especially beef) and egg yolks are strongly discouraged.

The Paleolithic Perspective

That cultures worldwide espouse consuming a predominantly plant-based diet that's supplemented minimally with animal-based foods should come as no surprise. After all, for millennia, our body adapted to, and thrived on, this inverse eating style. If we delve into the dietary life of our ancestors — who lived hundreds of thousands of years before our dietary wisdom evolved — we can learn still more about inverse eating and optimal foods. For although the American diet has changed drastically (becoming predominantly animal based and processed) during the twentieth century, our metabolism is still similar to what it was forty thousand years ago, as S. Boyd Eaton, M.D., coauthor of *The Paleolithic Prescription*, points out.

In this groundbreaking book, Dr. Eaton and colleagues detailed the eating habits and health status of both Paleolithic peoples and modern hunter-gatherer cultures. Using state-of-the-art assessment techniques, they explored the diet of humans who used stone tools during the Paleolithic Age. This was a period that began about 750,000 years ago and ended with the beginning of the Mesolithic Age, about 15,000 years ago. Because grains weren't cultivated and dairy products weren't consumed until about 11,000 years ago, the mainstay of our ancestors' diet was a large variety of wild vegetables (including many tubers), as well as wild game, such as deer, rabbit, or fowl. But this meat from wild game, with a fat content of about 4 percent, cannot compare to the 25 to 30 percent of fat found in the domesticated animal meat that most of us eat today (even lean cuts don't come close to 4 percent).

Indeed, with a plant/meat ratio of 65 percent plant food to 35 percent meat (and the intake of virtually no added salt, sugar, and of course, no processed food), we can ascertain that our Paleolithic ancestors naturally followed the same diet that is still espoused by most cultures and wisdom traditions today. And though Boyd points out that many of our ancestors succumbed to infectious diseases, it's believed that diet-linked ailments such as high blood pressure and heart disease were nonexistent in those societies. The key concept is that regardless of which part of the world you're viewing or how far back you go (tens of thousands of years to the Paleolithic Era or five thousand years to the evolution of Ayurveda), lean and low-fat inverse eating has prevailed.

Food as "Industrial Artifact"

We can always rely on our "fresh, whole food" past as a guide in choosing what to eat for optimal health today. If cultures have had a single dietary theme over the millennia, it's been to avoid tampering with the mystery, the "whole," the *chi* inherent in food and life. In a comment to me, this universal dietary truth was eloquently expressed by Hamid Algar, professor of Islamic Studies at the University of California, Berkeley.

Dr. Algar, a practitioner of Sufism, which is sometimes described as the aesthetic, mystical branch of Islam, said something that changed my view of food forever: "To treat food in a disrespectful fashion is ultimately disrespectful to the Qur'an . . . which tells us that food is sustenance that has been provided for us by Allah. Fast food, for instance, is the spiritual antithesis [of the dietary tenets of the Qur'an]." In other words, by "treating food as an industrial artifact that is consumed without any devotional context is to negate that food is a divine gift."

The words of one bumper sticker succinctly summarize this profound statement. It reads, "the best things in life aren't things." In other words, food isn't a "thing," merely an amalgam of objectively measured nutrients, the fuel to which we've reduced it; it's not an "industrial artifact." By denaturing food, we destroy what many religions see as the divine life force. We're not honoring food as the life-giving, life-containing gift that it is. And by eating refined food, we're also defiling something else: our bodies, yet another divine life-giving, life-containing gift.

My Denatured Food Diatribe

What does Dr. Algar mean by "industrial artifact"? He's referring to denatured or "dead" food — meaning that its life-giving nutrients have been removed or destroyed or that processing has created a food "product" far removed from its original state. In the United States, we use the terms *refined, adulterated,* and *processed* to describe food that's been much changed from its original form.

How does eating dead food translate into real life? It means you eat:

- more jam and apple pie than fresh fruit
- potato chips in lieu of baked potatoes
- enriched foods such as white bread, pasta, and rice instead of the whole-grain versions of these and other grains
- canned baked beans with ham in place of, say, freshly cooked beans
- fried and salted nuts or peanut butter in lieu of nuts and seeds in their shell
- highly processed meat, such as salami and bacon, instead of lean cuts of meat and poultry or fish
- more ice cream than yogurt
- lots of added oil instead of corn, sunflower seeds, olives, and so on

However you describe processed foods, they all have one thing in common: an unbalanced ratio of macronutrients (fat, carbohydrates, protein) and micronutrients (vitamins and minerals). By unbalanced, I'm referring to the change in the naturally occurring, inherent proportions of nutrients in food. Interestingly, even the water industry uses the terms *dead* or *empty* to describe water that's been stripped of its minerals.

Back in the U.S.A.

Most of us grew up having perhaps orange juice with bacon and eggs or super-sweet, highly processed cereal for breakfast — or even just a donut and coffee. Didn't lunch often consist of some kind of sandwich — perhaps bologna, salami, packaged ham and turkey, or canned tuna, sandwiched between white bread that'd been spread with mayonnaise and perhaps a small bit of lettuce and tomato? And wasn't it typical for many of us to have meat loaf or perhaps fried chicken for dinner, with some canned carrots and peas, white rice, or mashed potatoes? And in between meals, weren't many of us snacking (it seems endlessly) on soft drinks and munchies such as chips, cookies, and pastries?

In other words, aren't the majority of Americans more used to McDonald's than mustard greens, to Twinkies than tomatoes, and to frozen pizza than brown rice, steamed vegetables, and some fish or lean poultry? And doesn't the Standard American Diet lead us to label fresh, whole foods as "natural," "rabbit food," or "hippie food"? At the same time, we often link, sometimes with disdain, eating whole foods with food faddism, deprivation, or with being "good" (read "boring").

Not too long ago, the dietary powers that be in America caught on to the health benefits of consuming fresh, whole food, so much so that they changed the long-standing recommended four food groups that had reigned since the 1950s, the standard by which most of us were raised: 1) milk and dairy products; 2) meat, chicken, fish; 3) grains and breads; 4) and fruits and vegetables (and a fifth food group, consisting of sweets, alcohol, and fats). In April 1992, in response to the increase of heart disease and other diet-related ailments, the United States Department of Agriculture (USDA) created new dietary guidelines. These guidelines were presented in the form of a pyramid; called the Eating-Right Pyramid, this five-tiered graphic represents a diet that's strongly reminiscent of the Mediterranean diet and of Asian eating style. Can you guess how the tiers are arranged? If you guessed that the pyramid stresses plant-based food, with fewer servings of high-fat animal-based products and fat-dense processed foods, you're absolutely right.

Yet many of us still seem confused about this eating style, while others are resistant to following it. Indeed, a recent survey by the American Dietetic Association (ADA), which explored American food choices, concluded that 95 percent of us are knowledgeable about optimal foods and that more than 80 percent of adults are concerned about the effect of diet on future health. Yet despite this high level of knowledge and concern, "many individuals fail to apply their nutritional I.Q.," states the report. Astoundingly, only 8 percent of us have increased our intake of vegetables, and even fewer of us have upped our intake of fruits and fruit juices. The report concludes that "many Americans do not find eating pleasurable because they worry about fat, cholesterol, and weight gain, or feel guilty about eating the foods they enjoy."

Indeed, our emphasis on eating by number — weight watching, calorie counting, and figuring fat grams — has contributed to "orthorexia," a newly identified eating disorder that describes the growing number of us with obsessive fixations on eating the "right" food.

Health Benefits

To help you develop a broader perspective about the healing power of whole foods, I've provided a closer look at some of these nutrient-dense powerhouses and the benefits they bring. Designed to give you an overview of fresh, whole foods and their healing benefits, the following list is by no means exhaustive.

❧ *Have a phyto-feast.* In China, phytochemicals have been used for centuries to halt high blood pressure. In Europe, they've been linked with preventing lung cancer. In Japan, they're used as health enhancers. In America, scientists are exploring their ability to prevent common health problems, ranging from heart disease and cancer to high blood pressure, cataracts, and arthritis.

These naturally occurring substances in plant-based foods are being lauded as a "natural pharmacy" empowered with the ability to protect your health. Indeed, as research illuminates their potential health benefits, phytochemicals are emerging as the ultimate gift of health from Mother Nature. In fact, legumes and "colored" fruits and vegetables — such as spinach, carrots, cantaloupe, oranges, sweet potatoes, peppers, and tomatoes — may be especially effective disease fighters and a key to health and longevity.

❅ *"ACE" those antioxidants.* By now most of us know about antioxidants — protective nutrients such as beta-carotene and vitamins C and E (and lesser-known minerals, such as selenium and zinc) as well as some antioxidant-rich spices and herbs, such as turmeric. During the past decade, these star nutrients have received much press coverage because of their ability to protect your health by arresting the production of free radicals — toxins produced by cells in your body in reaction to, well, living (breathing, exercising) and to environmental factors such as air pollution. Left unchecked, free radicals can rob your health by damaging your cells. Over time, this process can leave you vulnerable to a plethora of health problems — from clogged arteries (atherosclerosis) to cataracts and cancer.

Putting a break on free radicals is easy if you include lots of antioxidant-rich foods in your diet. Which foods are these? You guessed it: fresh fruits and vegetables contain lots of vitamins A and C. Vitamin E is abundant in nuts and seeds (as well as in sweet potatoes), but if you eat too many nuts and seeds to get an adequate amount of vitamin E, you're sure to far surpass your daily allotment of fat. Instead, consider supplementing your fruit and vegetable intake with a supplement of between 100 to 400 I.U.'s daily.

❅ *Choose whole grains.* There's a big difference between whole grains and processed grains — not only in terms of the food itself, but also in terms of their effect on your health. Here's some background. During the industrial revolution of the mid-1850s, we learned to use huge cylinders to crush wheat kernels and separate out the (white) flour from the kernel's other parts — the wheat germ and bran. But as these separated foods — especially white flour — became inexpensive and plentiful, malnutrition became more widespread.

When it became clear that vitamins, minerals, and fiber were lacking in the processed products (such as white bread, white rice, and pasta), laws were passed requiring that the denatured food products be enriched. This meant that the few vitamins and minerals that we knew about at the time were to be added back into the refined product. These few nutrients didn't (and still don't) come close to the multitude of nutrients taken out (vitamins, minerals, fiber, enzymes, phytochemicals) that we know about today. In short, the whole of the edible plant is greater than the sum of the parts that have been added back. (Note: if a food label reads whole wheat, oats, rye, and so on, then the grain is still complete, with all its components and nutrients intact. If the label reads only *white* flour or *wheat* flour — without the word *whole* prefacing it — then the grain has been refined.)

❧ *Fill up with fiber.* Not too long ago, various media told us that pasta makes us fat. However, it would have been more accurate to say that eating lots of pasta made with refined white flour — minus the fiber — increases the likelihood of making you fat. Here's why. When you eat refined carbohydrates (such as white bread, white rice, sugar, jam) from which the fiber, germ, and other nutrients have been removed, your blood sugar (glucose) level rises. To metabolize the glucose, your body produces more insulin, a hormone (that is, chemical messenger).

Although the data is inconclusive, researchers believe that if you continually overload your body with refined foods — and with ensuing hits of high concentrations of glucose — your cells may eventually lose their ability to absorb the insulin. When this occurs, your cells become insulin resistant, increasing the odds of the glucose being stored as fat in the body. But when you eat complex carbohydrates (especially whole grains and legumes), with the fiber, germ, and nutrients still intact, your blood-sugar levels remain even, reducing the odds of producing too much glucose too soon and overtaxing your cells. The end result is that glucose is more likely to be metabolized and therefore less likely to be stored as fat.

❧ *Be bean wise.* There are literally hundreds of beans from which to choose, including heritage beans, some of which have been around for hundreds of years. Legumes offer a strong concentration of nutrients and often complement other whole foods —

especially whole grains — to make complete protein. Here's another reason to become bean wise: soybeans and minimally processed soy products such as tofu, soy burgers, tempeh, and soy milk offer a powerhouse of naturally occurring, disease-fighting substances that lower your risk of heart disease and some kinds of cancer.

Demystifying the Fats of Life

As you can see, fresh, whole, plant-based foods offer many health-enhancing benefits. But there's another key nutritional concept for you to consider for optimal health: fat. Perhaps more than any other nutrient, fat causes both concern and confusion.

No doubt about it — added fat (butter, margarine) and oil (liquid vegetable oils such as from corn and olives) are processed foods, industrial artifacts. Consider this: it takes an average of about two hundred ears of corn to process one cup of corn oil. Even if you're eating lots of whole foods to encourage optimal health, also cut back on added fat and oils, which, after all, aren't fresh, whole, or in their original, natural state.

What follows is a brief primer on fat. It's designed to give you the key concepts you'll need to demystify the profusion of confusion that surrounds fat in our diets.

≉ *Meet the "good" fats.* Virtually all food contains some fat. Yes, all food — even lettuce. For instance, one cup of iceberg lettuce, chopped, contains a minuscule 0.105 grams of fat. Want more proof? An orange has a measly 0.157 grams of fat; a cup of cooked oatmeal measures 2.3 grams; while a tablespoon of peanut butter contains 8 grams. Nature has figured out your fat intake for you: not only is naturally occurring fat a necessary nutrient, but you do need some fat for optimal health. Therefore, not only is it impossible to eat a completely fat-free diet, you wouldn't want to.

Contrary to popular belief, there is such a thing as fat that's good for you. Called essential fatty acids (EFAs), these fats are also known as omega-3s and omega-6s. They're essential because your body needs them to transport various vitamins (such as A, D, E, and K) through your body, keep your hair and skin healthy, help to lower blood cholesterol, boost your immune system, help you heal from cuts and wounds, and more. Because your body doesn't manufacture EFAs, you must get them through the foods you eat.

Essential fatty acids are found abundantly in high-fat, plant-based foods such as nuts, seeds, and processed liquid vegetable oils (like canola, corn, safflower, soy, and sesame), which are often referred to as polyunsaturated oils. However, when polyunsaturated oils are highly heated and processed to ensure a long shelf-life, most of the beneficial nutrients and good fats are processed out. The end result is that the balance (ratio) of omega 6s to omega 3s changes dramatically, with omega 6s far outweighing the omega 3s. Why should you care? Because, over time, consuming a disproportionally high intake of omega-6 fatty acids in processed oils may promote cancer, inflammation, and destructive changes in tissues.

Essentially, processing oil (even if it contains good fat) tampers with the natural balance of nutrients. Walnuts, flax seeds (ground into flax meal to make them more easily digestible), and fish (such as salmon and mackerel) contain lots of these good essential fats, in the ratio in which nature meant for you to consume them. To eat optimally, always strive to get these good fats from food rather than from processed oils.

❧ *Banish "bad" fats.* To solidify liquid vegetable oils into margarine, the liquid vegetable oils are "partially hydrogenated" (partially saturated with hydrogen atoms). This process creates unique molecules called trans-fatty acids, which do not exist naturally in the oils. Not only do trans-fats seem to raise blood levels of cholesterol and build-up in heart tissue, they also increase "bad," artery-clogging, LDL cholesterol, while decreasing the "good" HDL cholesterol that helps to whisk cholesterol out of your body. And more and more, trans-fats are being linked with an increased risk of certain cancers, such as breast cancer. Along with avoiding partially hydrogenated fat, to enhance health, avoid saturated fat, which stays hard at room temperature. Such fat is abundant in any animal-based food that isn't considered low fat, nonfat, or lean. Some examples are lard, butter, high-fat red meat, and processed meat, including bacon, salami, and ham.

Optimal Eating Strategies

By now it should be evident: the inverse eating style common worldwide is your key to optimal eating. In contrast, our typical diet, combined with our obsessive food analyzing, hasn't contributed to our health — physical or emotional. I'm proposing that in place of adding to your mighty arsenal of nutritional facts and figures, make the healing secret of optimal food your most-of-the-time eating style. As often as possible, eat fresh, whole foods in their natural state. Without an analytical, cognitive understanding of food, this strategy has helped humankind to continue as a species for hundreds of thousands of years, and as we've seen, it's still the way in which most (healthier) people eat throughout the world. Isn't it time we caught up with both the past and the present? What follows are some practical, simple optimal-eating strategies:

❧ *Eat inversely*. Consume mostly fresh, whole, plant-based foods in their natural state as often as possible. When you choose to eat animal-based foods, adopt an inverse-eating strategy: make fruits, vegetables, whole grains, and legumes your main meal, with meat, fowl, fish, or dairy serving as condiments. Another caveat: although most nuts and seeds are healthful, because they're high in fat, treat them, too, as a condiment. When having a meal — whether at home or while eating out — ask yourself if the main dish integrates these concepts. Try pasta primavera (noodles with vegetables); pizza with less (or no) cheese and more vegetables; have nachos with less cheese and more mashed beans.

❧ *Choose lean.* When consuming meat or dairy, let the exceptionally lean and low-fat animal foods on which we evolved be your guideline. To enhance health, select low-fat or nonfat dairy products and lean cuts of meat, skinless poultry, or fresh fish. As often as possible, avoid high-fat, high-sodium processed products such as ham, bacon, salami, or pastrami.

❧ *Get balanced.* Once you've decided on your baseline eating style, optimal, healthful eating also hinges on: 1) consuming adequate amounts of food each day from each food group; 2) cutting back on added fat — a little, a lot, or completely (how much you cut back on fat depends on whether your goal is to prevent a pending ailment or to reverse existing heart disease and; 3) consuming lots of naturally occurring — what you take in from your food — balanced vitamins, minerals, and enzymes.

❧ *Be nutrition wise.* Keep in mind that plant-based foods are low in sodium, calories, and fat (except for nuts and seeds); they contain absolutely no cholesterol; and they're high in disease-fighting antioxidants, phytochemicals, and fiber. Conversely, because animal-based foods are high in fat, high in cholesterol, relatively high in sodium and calories, and contain virtually no fiber, eat them in moderation or avoid them completely.

❧ *Limit nuts and seeds.* Fresh nuts and seeds are a good source of vitamin E and many minerals, including magnesium, which is needed for metabolizing calcium. Many are also a storehouse of unsaturated fatty acids needed for the production of energy, for growth, and stimulating the production of enzymes. But because they're exceptionally high in fat, eat them in moderation (perhaps a handful daily). Fresh nuts and seeds can add tasty, crunchy variety to vegetable and fruit salads, enhance the flavor and nutrient value of bean and grain dishes, or be enjoyed as a cholesterol-free snack.

❧ *Opt for Ornish.* If you have diagnosed heart disease — or are at high risk for developing it — consider following Dr. Dean Ornish's reversal diet (and entire program). Here are the general dietary guidelines. Every day consume fresh fruit (one to two servings a day); fresh vegetables (at least four servings a day); whole grains (at least six servings a day); and legumes (at least two servings a day). If desired, also have one cup of nonfat dairy product (such as milk, yogurt, and cottage cheese) and egg whites (one a day). Avoid or limit alcohol to two ounces a day; avoid or reduce added sugar or artificial sweeteners; limit sodium (if you have high blood pressure); avoid added oils or fat, nuts and seeds, avocados, olives, or coconut products; eat tofu in moderation. Although it has heart-healthy benefits, it is 49 percent fat. Choose the lower-fat variety whenever possible if you are concerned about heart disease.

❧ *Be creative.* It can be challenging at first to incorporate fresh, whole foods into your diet each day. To begin, decide which cuisine is your favorite. Chinese? Italian? Indian? Mexican? Thai? Then select a single, simple, plant-based recipe from your favorite cookbook or restaurant. If the recipe or dish calls for added oil or fat, cut the recommended amount in half (or omit it completely).

❧ *Eating-out strategies.* If you find yourself in a coffee shop or deli that seems to offer limited fare, ask the clerk what vegetables they do have on hand. It's likely that lettuce, tomato, and cucumber are available; sometimes even fresh mushrooms or olives are on hand. Consider using these ingredients as a base for a veggie-based sandwich or salad — with chicken or cheese on the side. Here's another easy-to-implement strategy: choose a sampling of plant-based appetizers for your main meal if most of the courses on the menu are mostly meat. When ordering cooked dishes, ask the waitperson to limit the amount of added fat or sauce. Then...enjoy!

Optimal Eating Recipe

The scene: Christmastime in Oslo, Norway, 1995. The concept: hosting a Christmas dinner in a restaurant for friends and colleagues, a Norwegian tradition. The characters: twenty-five people, some of whom do not know one another and an award-winning chef. The setting: a four-hundred-year-old building that has evolved into a restaurant. The challenge: to create an unforgettable gourmet Christmas meal of optimal foods (based on the inverse-eating concept).

The above scenario actually took place. I learned about it from the host of this incredible Christmas feast: my friend and colleague, Erik Ekker Solberg, a cardiologist, sports medicine specialist, and proud new papa who lives and works in Oslo. Personal preference and memory have a lot to do with what motivated Erik to turn vegetarian. Thirty years ago, this cardiologist became a vegetarian when he began a practice of yoga and meditation. "Over the years, I've noticed that I feel better, I'm not tired after eating, and it's easier to maintain the effects of meditation on a vegetarian diet. Feeling better and better, I wanted my friends to experience for themselves, firsthand, what I've been talking about, and just how fantastic such food can be."

He decided to create what in Norway is called *Julebord* ("Christmas table") with mostly plant-based foods. In the early 1990s, finding quality vegetarian meals in Norway was, at best, difficult. So Erik approached Norwegian culinary world champion chef, Bent Stiansen, who achieved this distinction when he was awarded the prestigious *Bocuse d'or* award in 1993. "We decided we could do better than most restaurants," says Erik. And they did.

Creating an incredible plant-based Christmas feast in Norway is no easy feat, especially because it goes against custom. Signaling the beginning of the season, as early as November, both home cooks and regional restaurants begin to serve Christmas fare, which typically includes fresh cod, halibut, or lutefisk; pork ribs and pork sausage patties in eastern Norway and dried mutton ribs on the West coast; rice porridge and rice cream served with a red fruit sauce are typical Christmas dinner desserts. Finding an abundance of fresh produce during the cold winter months can also be quite a challenge.

Enter award-winning chef Bent Stiansen, a world-renowned culinary artist who welcomes a challenge. Erik and Stiansen began to meet and plan the meal months before Christmas. Their goal was to come up with a menu consisting solely of fruits, vegetables, grains, legumes, and nuts and seeds, supplemented with dairy products. Other criteria were no eggs, no onion, no garlic (yogis consider onion and garlic stimulating and therefore an impediment to meditation), and no alcohol. "As we talked, Bent became inspired, as you might if you were planning to create a work of art," says Erik, who came up with the criteria. But it remained the chef's domain to make up the menu — which would be a surprise to both Erik and his guests. And what a surprise it was!

The extraordinary, unexpected starter was the two reserved rooms in Statholdergaarden, the restaurant in which the meal was served. When guests arrived, they immediately sensed the special scene that awaited them, both outside and in. Designated as the oldest building in Oslo (built in 1640), for centuries the building had housed the Bank of Norway. By the 1990s, it had become a top-of-the-line restaurant — with Bent Stiansen as its successful chef.

As each of the eight courses was served, Erik and his friends and colleagues were poised to savor and appreciate the ways in which Stiansen had interpreted the vegetarian guidelines he'd been given. They weren't disappointed. The fresh ingredients — purchased in Norway and from other European countries — released a bouquet of flavors that immediately earned their admiration. Examples include the first course, melon soup blended with other freshly squeezed juices and garnished with a sprig of green mint. Another favorite dish was the potato soup, prepared with high-quality almond potatoes, slight amounts of citrus and chili, and topped with croutons. The main dishes, served with an array of scintillating sauces, were also immensely appealing.

Stiansen called many of the lighter dishes "resting plates," because they were served between the more substantial dishes. All the while, only the chef knew the ingredients of the meal. What couldn't remain a secret, though, was the composition of each course, which was beautiful. Throughout the meal, the chef himself appeared before Erik and the guests to explain the food. During the evening, the explanations became an integral part of the ritual of the meal, a time to honor and bless the food.

As the meal progressed, there was much laughter; some guests gave speeches, while others enjoyed the exceptional atmosphere and company. But remember, this was an alcohol- and smoke-free feast! Instead of these "mood changers," the food, atmosphere, and other guests provided the stimulation. Erik describes the atmosphere as electrifying, a quality he attributes to the enthusiasm for the food that was experienced and expressed by the guests. After four and a half hours, the unforgettable meal ended.

"The ingredients were simple," says Erik. "It was the chef's artistry, rather than any unusual ingredients, that created the core flavoring in the food. His creativity and professionalism, and the regard and care in which he planned and prepared the food, turned potentially ordinary ingredients into a majestic, magical, memorable meal." The guests agree. Those who experienced the incredible eight-course vegetarian feast reflect that even though they'd eaten quite a bit, they didn't feel stuffed afterward. Rather, some told Erik that they felt "intoxicated." For others, eating over a period of four and a half hours had called for approaching the food in a somewhat meditative frame of mind: regarding one course after another; savoring the exceptional atmosphere; eating slowly; and with no alcoholic beverages, realizing that the excitement came from within.

As I listened to Erik describe his experience of the eventful meal, I realized that the feast was flavored with all the healing secrets of food. The key ingredient was the inverse-eating concept in action: fruits, vegetables, grains, legumes, nuts and seeds, and some dairy foods. And there was the pleasure of sharing food with friends; feeling fine throughout the evening; bringing a meditative mindfulness to the meal; and appreciating the culinary artistry.

Those who attended Erik's unique *Julebord* encouraged him to replicate it. And so he does, some years, although now Erik is the chef, and he cooks an incredible Christmas feast for friends at his home. "Last year, I invited twelve friends over, and served six courses," he says. Erik talks about the wonderful sense of connection that's created: "With no alcohol, the intoxication comes from the inner spirit," suggests Erik. "When you cook for others in this way, you're offering a gift of love through the food. It's always a great evening."

PART THREE

The Healing Secrets in Action

chapter eight

The Meal Meditation

After all, there's no need
to say anything
at first. An orange, peeled
and quartered, flares
like a tulip on a Wedgwood plate.
Anything can happen.
Outside the sun
has rolled up her rugs
and night strewn salt
across the sky. My heart
is humming a tune
I haven't heard in years!
Quiet's cool flesh —
let's sniff and eat it.
There are ways
to make of the moment
a topiary
so the pleasure's in
walking through.

"Flirtation" by Rita Dove

In this chapter, you are cordially invited to join me in the meal
meditation. As you do, you'll become empowered to experience
food as the symphonic masterpiece that it is, that plays the notes of

all the healing secrets of food discussed in this book: socializing, feelings, mindfulness, appreciation, connection, and optimal food. To help us eat with all-encompassing awareness is one of the major intentions of the meal meditation, a culmination of everything we've learned so far in this book.

"When we meditate," explains psychologist and Taoist meditator Michael Mayer, "we feel connected to ourselves, others, and the universe itself." Over thousands of years, practitioners have developed simple but powerful techniques that enrich this connection by focusing mind, body, soul, and our subtle energy. The meal meditation consists of two time-honored techniques — mudras (hand gestures) and mantras (repeated phrases) — that will enable you to more effectively cultivate and integrate the healing secrets into your daily menu. These mudras and mantras may be practiced independent of or before the meal meditation, which I will describe for you step-by-step in the final section of this chapter.

The meal meditation will show you how to use particular hand mudras that empower you to spice food with appreciative, loving, meditative awareness. In addition, the following meditative phrases (mantras) may further enhance your dining experience. Based on your personal preference, consider practicing the three elements of the meal meditation — mudras, mantras, and the meditation itself — silently or perhaps with some serene music that encourages the meditative mood to wrap itself around you. One caveat: as you weave together the moments of the meal meditation, the rest of the world must wait.

Making Mudras

In Islam, a muezzin is a Muslim crier who calls the faithful to prayer. Over the centuries, mudras — hand and body gestures that are believed to channel energy in the body and breath — have evolved to call the meditator silently to a deeper experience of meditation.

In the West, the most familiar mudra is the gesture of veneration. Hands placed together in front of the chest, palms touching, fingertip to fingertip: this is a traditional gesture of respect and devotion that has become the very emblem of prayer. In Eastern traditions, deities themselves are sometimes portrayed making this gesture to venerate higher gods. Buddhas are often represented making various hand gestures, based on their particular attributes. For instance, the traditional meditation mudra entails placing the top of one hand in the palm of the other, then placing the semicupped hands on the lap. Another mudra is extending one hand downward with the palm open facing forward; this is a gesture of giving, signifying the granting of a blessing. And bringing the tips of the thumbs and forefingers together, while keeping the other fingers straight, is a gesture of exposition and teaching; called the *Chin mudra* by yogis, this gesture is believed to release energy in the lower abdomen and back.

"Most of us take these hand and body gestures for granted," writes psychologist and yoga practitioner Richard C. Miller in *Yoga Journal*. Not only do they "influence the way we experience our breath and energy *(prana)* during... prayer, blessing, and meditation," mudras also "help us enter more deeply into meditation."

Meaningful Mantras

Imagine that you are preparing food for your family. As you cook, your thoughts float from one topic to another: an impending deadline, taxes, visitors you're expecting next week, next month's vacation plans, and so on. Distracted, you suddenly knock over a glass, then spend the next few minutes sweeping up the broken pieces and vacuuming up any remaining slivers. Feeling frustrated, you realize you dropped the glass because you were distracted. How do you avoid this type of scenario? Become more aware of what you're doing. To accomplish this, you repeat the phrase "I remain focused on the food" both silently to yourself and sometimes out loud as you prepare the rest of the meal. Such a repeated phrase is called a mantra.

Georg Feuerstein, in *The Shambhala Guide to Yoga*, describes mantras as "a power-charged form of thought that serves as an instrument of spiritual liberation." Remaining in the moment by repeating a phrase is an age-old tradition. For instance, devout yogis and Hindus developed mantras to replace helter-skelter thoughts and emotions with focused meditative attention on a particular object. Jews turn to *berakhot,* or blessings, to substitute free-floating feelings with a state of appreciative and compassionate connection. For Christians, prayers serve as expressions of focused thoughts, hopes, or needs. Buddhists connect to an awareness beyond the limited self through the practice of *metta* (loving kindness) as well as through meditative chanting. Muslims concentrate their minds, hearts, and spirits with both prayer *(salat)* and food-focused manners *(adab)* that encourage a connection to God consciousness *(taqwa)* each time they eat. And more recently, the word *affirmation,* meaning a spoken or silent phrase you focus on to achieve a desired outcome, has entered the popular lexicon.

Whether through repeated phrases, blessings, prayers, chanting, affirmations, or specific meal-related manners and practices — appreciative, meditative words filled with loving intention have stood at the center of human endeavors — including dining — for ages.

Sacred Words

What follows is a concise compilation of some mantras, blessings, prayers, words of thankfulness, and affirmations, as well as "consciousness concepts," all of which provide a way to focus and integrate appreciative thoughts during the meal meditation. Repeat a thought or phrase until your thoughts become focused on your food. Or, as you read these various phrases and concepts, consider keeping notes to create your own food-focused meditative phrases. The process begins with your curiosity, but because the reward is being in the moment itself, there is no goal or destination other than the ultimate gift of connection to the beneficent Mother Nature, who makes all meals possible.

Mantras

- *Om* (a sacred Sanskrit syllable).
- *Seventy-two labors brought us this food. We should know how*

it comes to us (excerpt from a Buddhist chant).

- *May eating help me to open to the true nature of life* (metta).

Blessings

- *Bless this food before me and all those who brought it to my table* (simple Hindu grace).
- *Blessed art Thou, O Lord our God, Creator of the Universe, Who brings forth bread from the earth* (the Moszi, the Jewish blessing over bread).
- *Dear Heavenly Father, bless this food for the nourishment of our bodies* (Christian grace said by Jerry Scherwitz).

Prayers

- *Beloved Mother Nature, you are here on our table as our food. You are endless, bountiful, benefactress of all. Please grant us health and strength, wisdom and dispassion to find permanent peace and joy* (ancient Sanskrit prayer).
- *Praise to thee, oh God, for allowing us to eat, drink, and be satisfied with the food and the liquid* (excerpt from an Islamic prayer said after eating).
- *Holy God, as you feed me spiritually with the Eucharist, remind me of the . . . love of Jesus* (Christian prayer said by Father Robert Bryant).

Thanks

- *We are thankful for the triumph of soul food, "black folk cooking." Spiced with spirit and served from the heart, it transforms body and soul and helps the spirit soar* (inspired by a quote from soul food restaurateur Pamela Strobel).
- *I honor the life you have given so that I may be fed. I am*

thankful for the great gift you have given me this day. My heart is full for the sacrifice you have made. I respect your offering and so will waste no part of your gift. My spirit bows to your spirit (Anasazi "Meal Thanksgiving," from *Ancient Echoes* by Mary Summer Rain).

- *Lord be with us on this day of thanksgiving. Help us make the most of this life we are living. As we are about to partake of this bountiful meal, let us not forget the needy and the hunger they feel. Help us to show compassion in all that we do. And for all our many blessings we say thank you* ("Thanksgiving Blessings," from *Graces* by Helen Latham).

Affirmations

Here are some affirmations I've used:

- *As I eat, I open my heart to feelings of love, joy, and peace.*
- *When I approach food with gratitude, I enjoy it more.*
- *More and more, I open my senses to the delights of food: its colors, fragrances, tastes, and textures.*

Consciousness Concepts

- *Eating food quickly or gulping down liquids, without conscious or reverential recognition of the nourishment, is to treat food disrespectfully. Chewing slowly, with awareness, represents a conscious understanding that the food is being provided by God* (Islamic etiquette).
- *Food is a physical "bridge" between humans (earthly consciousness) and the gods (heavenly spirits). It is the vehicle whereby loving intentions and actions can be communicated to the gods and, in turn, reflected back to people via good fortune* (Chinese ancient folk tradition).
- *Slow down life and create the unhurried, authentic experience of a tea ritual by becoming a* chajin, *a person of "tea mind." As*

much as it is an actual ceremony, the Way of Tea is also a con-
sciousness, a "mentality of elegance," an ability to appreciate
the beauty of the elements — from the singing of the water as
it is poured, to the ebb and flow of the human voice during con-
versation (inspired by a conversation with David Lee
Hoffman, proprietor of Silk Road Teas).

The Meal Meditation

The Meal Meditation that follows will enable you to practice, internalize, and integrate all the healing secrets of food as well as the
mudras and mantras discussed above. Each time you practice
the meal meditation, you'll be metabolizing the ultimate "multiple
vitamin," one that holds the power to nourish not only your physical health but also your social, emotional, and spiritual well-being.
As you get better at weaving together each moment of the meditation, consider using it whenever you're involved in any food-
related activity — from planting and harvesting to planning a meal,
shopping, eating, digesting, or doing dishes.

⅔ ***Begin by relaxing.*** To start the heart dance between you
and your food, position yourself the same way each time you dine.
You may prefer to fold your hands gently in your lap; or perhaps
you'll want to place them on the table or to let your arms hang comfortably at your side. Whatever position you choose, over time it
will become a gentle reminder that leads you into the meditation.
Now simply relax by inhaling deeply, then exhale slowly and completely. Do this three times, with your eyes closed or focused on
your food.

⅔ ***Visualize.*** Next, envision a ball of liquid golden light several inches above your head. Then imagine it melting, then flowing
through your head, then down through your shoulders and to your
arms and hands, then through your heart and torso, then down
your legs and to your feet.

⅔ ***Create a mudra.*** Continuing to envision golden light emanating from your body — especially from your heart center and

hands — position your hands as if there were a small beach ball hovering just over your food and your hands are holding that beach ball. As you do this, direct positive feelings into your heart center.

❧ *Choose optimal foods.* Holding love and appreciation in your heart, and remaining free of judgment, focus on what you are eating. Is the food in front of you fresh and whole? Does the meal consist mostly of fresh, whole vegetables, fruits, grains, beans and peas, and small servings of nuts and seeds, with (optional) lean, low-fat, smaller portions of fish, poultry, meat, or dairy foods? Or is your meal predominantly processed food products, consisting, for instance, of white bread, mayonnaise, a hamburger, pizza, or French fries? Are you snacking — without awareness — mostly on prepackaged pies and cookies, or have you chosen instead to snack on a fruit smoothie, a handful of nuts, or your favorite bread? In other words, have you taken the time to choose food that is a positive life force, a nurturer, a gift that recharges and sustains?

❧ *Unite socially.* If you are dining with others, envision a ray or thread of the golden liquid connecting your heart center to the heart center of the other person or people at the table. If you're alone, connect the golden thread to the silent players responsible for bringing the food to the table — the cook, grocer, farmer, waiter — whether or not you know them. Or link it to an image (such as a photograph) or memory of a person, or people, you love.

❧ *Tune in to your feelings.* Continuing to relax and breathe deeply, identify how you are feeling. First, are you feeling hungry? And if so, how hungry: a little, somewhat, or a lot? Use this knowledge to make a decision about how much or how little you want to eat. Also, do you still feel filled with positive, loving emotions? Or before eating (or shopping, cooking, digesting), do you still need to release painful emotions, such as anger and anxiety?

Throughout the meal, continue the internal dance between your feelings and the food you are eating. Check in every five minutes or so to decide if you are still feeling hungry or are now feeling comfortably satiated, or perhaps even stuffed. Because it takes about twenty minutes for your mind/body to register the effects of food (such as feeling more relaxed, calm, or alert), continue the invisible feeling-food dialogue to decide if those carbohydrates have calmed you down, the high-fat food has made you feel "foggy," or the protein has perked you up.

❧ *Practice mindfulness.* Eating mindfully includes being aware of all the healing secrets of food. All the while, the senses play a significant part in helping you to remain meditative. Look at the food in front of you. "Taste" the colors first. Are they muted, bright? Is there a lot of food, or are portions small? What about the fragrance of the food: does it smell sweet or sour? When you get in close to sniff, what temperature do you sense: hot, warm, or cold? As you continue to hold your hands in the ball mudra over the food, are they becoming warmer or colder? What kinds of sounds surround you? Clinking glasses, pouring water, the lull of soft conversation? Is there much movement and noise, or are you and your companions calm and quiet? Have the utensils and napkins been laid out for you? If so, by whom?

Continue to focus mindfully on the food and environs throughout your meal, adding the sounds of chewing, the texture of the food, the way in which the scent of the food changes as you chew, how your tongue and teeth prepare the food to be swallowed, the different tastes that envelop your mouth, and any other dining sensations that may enter your awareness before, during, and after eating.

❧ *Be appreciative.* Now think of a person you love or especially like, or visit (in your memory) a place or event that you have found particularly pleasing. As you continue to inhale deeply, bring these positive, loving feelings into your heart center and release any negative thoughts, feelings, or tension with each slow, long exhalation.

Continuing to hold the ball mudra while remaining in a state of calm, relaxed appreciation — for a person or place, or especially for the food before you — express your gratitude with a mantra, blessing, prayer, thanks, affirmation, or consciousness concept. Or simply shoot a quick "arrow prayer" to the food with a brief, sincere thank you.

❧ *Create connection.* Connecting with food calls for evoking loving intention and then projecting it onto the food. To do this, focus again on the golden energy flowing through you and on the appreciative, loving feelings you are holding in your heart. As your hands continue to surround both sides of the dish, through visualization, project rays of this golden light into your food. Do this by imagining a pulsating glow of light going from your heart center into the food; then imagine an amorphous mist that spreads like golden, tiny bits of speckled fog from the palms of your hands into the food. In this way, you flavor food with love.

Now, feeling relaxed and calm, with awareness of your social environment and your feelings, with mindfulness, appreciation, with a sense of loving connection in your heart, and nonjudgmental attention on your food, it is time to begin the extraordinary experience of eating.

postscript

Nutritional technology may have changed over the years, but the needs of our souls have not. What greater gifts can we give to ourselves than to let food nourish us multidimensionally each time we eat, to experience the essential qualities of our being through food's power to heal socially, emotionally, spiritually, and physically?

Each of the healing secrets of food is imbued with ancient food wisdom that has sustained us for millennia. I believe these secrets are a template, a time-tested set of nutritional guidelines that create a clear picture about not only what to eat but how to eat and also how to live: consciously, filled with a sense of wonder inherent in the alchemical union between human beings and food — one of life's vital, elemental elixirs.

As nutritional science continues to evolve, I advise you to consider the nutritional data gleaned from our evolutionary and spiritual ancestors and from current research, then to draw your own conclusions about the best way to eat. For, today more than ever, you can make smart choices about how you eat and live that will help lower your risk not only of heart disease but of many types of cancer, adult-onset diabetes, high blood pressure, obesity, a weakened immune system, and a plethora of other food-related health problems.

Having read this book, now you have even more health-wise choices. You can look to food as more than medicine, perceiving it as the symphonic masterpiece that it is, capable of bringing pleasure to your palate and satisfaction to your soul. And instead of depending solely on scientific studies, you can rely on your own judgment and consciousness to digest the healing secrets of food revealed throughout this book.

In place of spending the precious life that you've been given counting calories, you can choose instead to enjoy life and food by dining with others; being aware of the food-mood connection; appreciating food and its origins — from the heart; eating mindfully and nonjudgmentally; flavoring food with love; and eating fresh, whole foods in their natural state. And you can practice these secrets as often as is realistically possible rather than regarding them as the perfect eating style to be followed rigidly and religiously.

Implementing the healing secrets of food calls for blending your own ingredients for success: abundant curiosity, an understanding of integrative eating and optimal foods, and a willingness to merge your personal health goals with ancient food wisdom and the latest science. Then you may access food's invisible power to sustain, rejuvenate, and heal — and in the process, find true nourishment.

appendix

Your Integrative Eating Profile

Where are you now? After having read *The Healing Secrets of Food*, it's a good time to check in by using Your Integrative Eating Profile. This profile is not a quiz. It's not an assessment. It's not a measure of good or bad, right or wrong, pass or fail, perfect or imperfect. Rather, I created the following profile as your personal "consciousness-raising" guide, a reflective tool designed to give you an indication of how much or how little you're integrating the social, psychological, spiritual, and biological healing secrets of food into your everyday eating patterns.

When I taught the healing secrets at California Pacific Medical Center's Institute of Health and Healing in San Francisco and lectured about them at San Francisco State University's Department of Holistic Health, I gave course participants the profile both before and after the course. Having the participants fill out the profile before they've learned about the healing secrets provides me with a baseline perspective of their integrative eating status before the course begins. Looking over the profile afterward reveals the degree to which they've made the changes necessary to pursue their personal nutrition or health goals. In this light, consider the profile as a lighthouse that helps you to get your bearings, a guide to help you determine your nutrition whereabouts so that you can choose the nutritional paths that are optimal for you.

Checking the Checkpoints

Your Integrative Eating Profile provides a bevy of benefits. Once you check off the boxes and tally your total score, not only will you have a clearer perspective of the integrative eating areas in which you're strong, but you'll also have a better understanding of areas you may want to improve. Another benefit: reviewing the profile will empower you with a new slew of health-enhancing integrative eating strategies.

❧ *Tallying your scores.* To reap the rewards, complete each social, psychological, spiritual, and biological food questionnaire below by checking the boxes that best represent your current eating style. As you fill out the profile, please note that each questionnaire has two sections: score the top section by tallying all the plus (+) numbers; tally the bottom section by adding all the minus (-) numbers. Then subtract the minus subtotal from the plus subtotal and enter the results on the total line at the bottom of each profile.

❧ *Interpreting your scores.* At the bottom of each profile, you'll find a nutrition scoring key that tells you if your social, psychological, spiritual, and biological nutrition scores rank as "excellent," "good," "satisfactory," or "needs improvement." To discover your total integrative eating score for all four sections, add the totals from each of the four profiles; then read about the interpretation of your total score at the end of the profile.

Social Nutrition
PERSONAL PROFILE

For each question, check every box in the column that best
represents your food-related social dynamic.

	Never 0	Rarely +1	Sometimes +2	Usually +3	Almost Always +4	Always +5
1. I eat with:						
coworkers	❑	❑	❑	❑	❑	❑
friends	❑	❑	❑	❑	❑	❑
family members	❑	❑	❑	❑	❑	❑

2. I eat at home at the dining table.

	❑	❑	❑	❑	❑	❑

3. The social atmosphere in which I prepare food is:

	Never 0	Rarely +1	Sometimes +2	Usually +3	Almost Always +4	Always +5
serene	❑	❑	❑	❑	❑	❑
pleasing	❑	❑	❑	❑	❑	❑
fun	❑	❑	❑	❑	❑	❑

4. While dining, I consider my surroundings.

	❑	❑	❑	❑	❑	❑

5. I eat homemade meals.

	❑	❑	❑	❑	❑	❑

Subtotal + _____

	Never	Rarely	Sometimes	Usually	Almost Always	Always
	0	-1	-2	-3	-4	-5

6. I eat meals from:

fast-food outlets	❏	❏	❏	❏	❏	❏
delicatessens and supermarkets	❏	❏	❏	❏	❏	❏

7. I eat by myself.

	❏	❏	❏	❏	❏	❏

8. When I eat, I am:

walking, rushing	❏	❏	❏	❏	❏	❏
at my desk at work	❏	❏	❏	❏	❏	❏
in my car	❏	❏	❏	❏	❏	❏
at my computer	❏	❏	❏	❏	❏	❏
watching TV	❏	❏	❏	❏	❏	❏
reading	❏	❏	❏	❏	❏	❏
talking on the phone	❏	❏	❏	❏	❏	❏
driving	❏	❏	❏	❏	❏	❏

9. The social atmosphere in which I prepare food is:

hectic	❏	❏	❏	❏	❏	❏
tense	❏	❏	❏	❏	❏	❏
bland/boring	❏	❏	❏	❏	❏	❏

Subtotal – _____

Total Social Nutrition Score: (+) or (-) _____

+22 and over	*Excellent*
+6 to +21	*Good*
–10 to +5	*Satisfactory*
–11 and below	*Needs Improvement*

Psychological Nutrition
PERSONAL PROFILE

*For each question, check every box in the column
that best represents your food-related feelings.*

	Never	Rarely	Sometimes	Usually	Almost Always	Always
	0	+1	+2	+3	+4	+5

1. Before eating, I check my hunger level.

| ❑ | ❑ | ❑ | ❑ | ❑ | ❑ |

2. I eat only when I am hungry.

| ❑ | ❑ | ❑ | ❑ | ❑ | ❑ |

3. After eating, I feel comfortably full.

| ❑ | ❑ | ❑ | ❑ | ❑ | ❑ |

4. After eating, I feel:

	Never	Rarely	Sometimes	Usually	Almost Always	Always
relaxed	❑	❑	❑	❑	❑	❑
calm	❑	❑	❑	❑	❑	❑
alert	❑	❑	❑	❑	❑	❑

Subtotal + _____

	Never	Rarely	Sometimes	Usually	Almost Always	Always
	0	-1	-2	-3	-4	-5

5. After eating, I feel stuffed.

❏ ❏ ❏ ❏ ❏ ❏

6. I feel anxious about the "best" way to eat.

❏ ❏ ❏ ❏ ❏ ❏

7. I have food cravings.

❏ ❏ ❏ ❏ ❏ ❏

8. I eat because I feel:

depressed	❏	❏	❏	❏	❏	❏
sad	❏	❏	❏	❏	❏	❏
anxious	❏	❏	❏	❏	❏	❏
angry	❏	❏	❏	❏	❏	❏
frustrated	❏	❏	❏	❏	❏	❏
happy	❏	❏	❏	❏	❏	❏

9. I feel good or righteous when I eat what I think I should.

❏ ❏ ❏ ❏ ❏ ❏

10. When I overeat, I feel:

bad	❏	❏	❏	❏	❏	❏
guilty	❏	❏	❏	❏	❏	❏
gluttonous	❏	❏	❏	❏	❏	❏

Subtotal – _____

Total Psychological Nutrition Score: (+) or (-) _____

+11 and over	Excellent
–1 to +10	Good
–14 to –2	Satisfactory
–15 and below	Needs Improvement

Spiritual Nutrition
PERSONAL PROFILE

*For each question, check every box in the column that best represents
your degree of mindfulness, appreciation, and connection to food.*

	Never 0	Rarely +1	Sometimes +2	Usually +3	Almost Always +4	Always +5

1. I plan and prepare meals:

	Never 0	Rarely +1	Sometimes +2	Usually +3	Almost Always +4	Always +5
with care	❑	❑	❑	❑	❑	❑
with appreciation	❑	❑	❑	❑	❑	❑

2. I express gratitude for food through prayer, blessings, heartfelt thankfulness.

	Never 0	Rarely +1	Sometimes +2	Usually +3	Almost Always +4	Always +5
	❑	❑	❑	❑	❑	❑

3. Before and during eating, I focus on the food's:

	Never 0	Rarely +1	Sometimes +2	Usually +3	Almost Always +4	Always +5
color	❑	❑	❑	❑	❑	❑
aroma	❑	❑	❑	❑	❑	❑
portion size	❑	❑	❑	❑	❑	❑
flavor(s)	❑	❑	❑	❑	❑	❑

4. I eat with my senses, by:
appreciating

	Never 0	Rarely +1	Sometimes +2	Usually +3	Almost Always +4	Always +5
the presentation	❑	❑	❑	❑	❑	❑
tasting textures	❑	❑	❑	❑	❑	❑
savoring scents	❑	❑	❑	❑	❑	❑

5. I focus solely on food and the experience of dining.

	Never 0	Rarely +1	Sometimes +2	Usually +3	Almost Always +4	Always +5
	❑	❑	❑	❑	❑	❑

Continued on next page

	Never	Rarely	Sometimes	Usually	Almost Always	Always
	0	+1	+2	+3	+4	+5

6. I appreciate the web of humanity (farmers, grocers, cooks) surrounding food.

| ❑ | ❑ | ❑ | ❑ | ❑ | ❑ |

7. I consider the elements of nature that create food.

| ❑ | ❑ | ❑ | ❑ | ❑ | ❑ |

8. I eat with loving regard for food.

| ❑ | ❑ | ❑ | ❑ | ❑ | ❑ |

9. I honor the mystery of life in food.

| ❑ | ❑ | ❑ | ❑ | ❑ | ❑ |

10. After eating, I:

	Never	Rarely	Sometimes	Usually	Almost Always	Always
savor the moment	❑	❑	❑	❑	❑	❑
reflect on the meal	❑	❑	❑	❑	❑	❑

Subtotal + _____

	Never	Rarely	Sometimes	Usually	Almost Always	Always
	0	-1	-2	-3	-4	-5

11. I concentrate on, or think about, work, chores, etc., while eating.
❑ ❑ ❑ ❑ ❑ ❑

12. I judge others by what they eat.
❑ ❑ ❑ ❑ ❑ ❑

13. I eat quickly.
❑ ❑ ❑ ❑ ❑ ❑

14. After eating, I get up and get going.
❑ ❑ ❑ ❑ ❑ ❑

15. After eating, I wash the dishes begrudgingly.
❑ ❑ ❑ ❑ ❑ ❑

Subtotal – _____

Total Spiritual Nutrition Score: (+) or (-) _____

+63 and over *Excellent*
+43 to +62 *Good*
+24 to +42 *Satisfactory*
+23 and below *Needs Improvement*

Biological Nutrition
PERSONAL PROFILE

*For each question, check the box that best represents
your relationship to food.*

	Never 0	Rarely +1	Sometimes +2	Usually +3	Almost Always +4	Always +5
1. I eat fresh:						
fruits	❑	❑	❑	❑	❑	❑
vegetables	❑	❑	❑	❑	❑	❑
whole grains	❑	❑	❑	❑	❑	❑
legumes	❑	❑	❑	❑	❑	❑
nuts	❑	❑	❑	❑	❑	❑
seeds	❑	❑	❑	❑	❑	❑

```
Subtotal + _____
```

	Never 0	Rarely -1	Sometimes -2	Usually -3	Almost Always -4	Always -5
2. I eat food that is:						
fast *(such as McDonald's)*	❑	❑	❑	❑	❑	❑
processed *(canned, packaged)*	❑	❑	❑	❑	❑	❑
prepared *(deli, take-out)*	❑	❑	❑	❑	❑	❑
sweet *(donuts, muffins)*	❑	❑	❑	❑	❑	❑
fried *(potato chips, fried chicken)*	❑	❑	❑	❑	❑	❑

Continued on next page

	Never	Rarely	Sometimes	Usually	Almost Always	Always
	0	-1	-2	-3	-4	-5

3. I overeat.

❏ ❏ ❏ ❏ ❏ ❏

4. I undereat.

❏ ❏ ❏ ❏ ❏ ❏

5. I try different diets.

❏ ❏ ❏ ❏ ❏ ❏

6. I count calories, fat grams, and so on.

❏ ❏ ❏ ❏ ❏ ❏

7. I obsess about food.

❏ ❏ ❏ ❏ ❏ ❏

Subtotal – _____

Total Biological Nutrition Score: (+) or (-) _____

+14 and over   *Excellent*
+3 to +13   *Good*
–8 to +2   *Satisfactory*
–9 and below   *Needs Improvement*

Your Integrative Eating Score

To find your total integrative eating score, add up the total scores for each of the four sections, then enter it below.

Total Integrative Eating Score: _____

Evaluating your score:

+110 or over *(excellent):*
You are eating optimally and integratively most of the time. Both what and how you eat are optimal — not only for your health but also for the quality of your life.

+51 to +109 *(good):*
The foods you choose, and how you eat, are both fairly good. You eat optimally sometimes; when you're not able to — or choose not to — you let it go.

-8 to +50 *(satisfactory):*
Food and eating are often issues for you. Either you're not sure how to make better choices about what and how to eat or doing so hasn't been a priority for you. Your food choices and approach to food are fairly typical, which leaves lots of room for making beneficial changes.

-9 and below *(needs improvement):*
Your eating style is far from optimal or integrative. Decide if you want to take steps toward eating integratively. Once you have the intention to do so, get some ideas for how to begin by reviewing the practical tips at the end of each healing secret chapter, or look over the questions in each section of Your Integrative Eating Profile for some easy-to-implement suggestions.

acknowledgments

I am eternally grateful to all those who have contributed to the rich repository of food wisdom that has evolved over the centuries.

To friends, family, colleagues, and students who have "flavored" *The Healing Secrets of Food* with their own rich repertoires, reflections, skills, and support, I extend heartfelt gratitude:

To my husband, Larry, who first conceived of the healing secrets of food early one morning — then shared them with me; who has lived the concepts in this book from their inception; and who has encouraged me and provided editorial insight throughout the entire research and writing process.

To Stephen Sparler, longtime colleague and friend, for being the first reader; for his editorial input, critical thinking, and for contributing his spiritual food views.

To friends, especially the literary Linda Gibbs, who generously shared her insights about a meal she had in my home; to David Leivick, whose description of his pizza odyssey — and his passion for and appreciation of fantastic, fresh food in general — enhanced the chapter on mindfulness; to premier publicist Isabella Michon; and like-minded colleagues: to brilliant beat author and poet Brenda Knight, and to nutrition and food aficionados Amy Bacheller and Sarah Ellis.

To friend Nischala Devi, who "grocked" my work early on and

graciously shared inspirational insights about yogic nutrition.

To Ed Espe Brown, for providing pearls of wisdom about Buddhism, food, and eating.

To others who shared their unique food views: visionary, innovator, and scholar Larry Dossey; Effie Chow, who helps and inspires so many with her "whole-person medical Qigong" systems approach; and Rabbi Harold Schulweis, who has the unique ability to wax poetic about Judaism's refined food consciousness and its commitment to compassion.

To Jodie and Tim Wedgwood, friends from England who are radio broadcasters; thank you for some fine suggestions.

To my literary agent, Patti Breitman, for her support...always and for her vision of the book.

To New World Library editorial director Georgia A. Hughes, for her excellent insights and suggestions; it is an honor and pleasure to work with her.

To Judith Tolson, who invited me to teach workshops on the healing secrets of food at California Pacific Medical Center's Institute of Health and Healing in San Francisco.

To psychologist Jay Azarow, who opened the door to his classroom at San Francisco State University and encouraged me to lecture in his "Holistic Health: Western Perspectives" course.

To the many people who have attended my workshops and lectures; your feedback and enthusiasm have been inspirational.

And to all those, who by living the healing secrets of food, continue to contribute to the stream of wisdom about the ancient human longing to find meaning in food and drink.

selected bibliography

Achterberg, Jeanne. *Rituals of Healing: Using Imagery for Health and Wellness.* New York: Bantam Books, 1994.

Benson, Herbert. *Timeless Healing: The Power and Biology of Belief.* New York: Fireside, 1996.

Benson, Herbert, and William Proctor. *Beyond the Relaxation Response.* New York: Times Books, 1984.

Borysenko, Joan. *Minding the Body, Mending the Mind.* Reading, MA: Addison-Wesley, 1987.

Brillat-Savarin, Jean Anthelme. *The Physiology of Taste.* New York: Knopf, 1949.

Brown, Ed Espe. *Tomato Blessings and Radish Teachings: Recipes and Reflections.* New York: Riverhead Books, 1997.

Buber, Martin. *I and Thou.* New York: Scribner, 1958.

Capra, Fritjof. *The Tao of Physics.* New York: Bantam, 1984.

Chopra, Deepak. *Ageless Body, Timeless Mind: The Quantum Alternative to Growing Old.* New York: Harmony Books, 1993.

Chuk, Stephan, and Carol and Charles Wong. *Mooncakes and Hungry Ghosts: Festivals of China.* San Francisco: China Books and Periodicals, 1991.

Counihan, Carole, and Penny Van Esterik, eds. *Food and Culture: A Reader.* New York: Routledge, 1997.

David, Marc. *Nourishing Wisdom*. New York: Bell Tower, 1991.

Devi, Nischala. *The Healing Path of Yoga: Alleviate Stress, Open Your Heart, and Enrich Your Life*. New York: Three Rivers Press, 2000.

Dossey, Larry. *Healing Words*. San Francisco: HarperCollins, 1993.

_____. *Prayer Is Good Medicine*. San Francisco: HarperCollins, 1996.

_____. *Space, Time, and Medicine*. Boston: Shambhala, 1982.

Douglas, Mary. *Purity and Danger: An Analysis of the Concepts of Pollution and Taboo*. London: Routledge, 1966.

Feuerstein, George, and Stephan Bodian, eds. *Living Yoga: A Comprehensive Guide for Daily Life*. New York: Tarcher/Putnam, 1993.

Fisher, M. F. K. *Dubious Honors*. San Francisco: North Point Press, 1988.

Gawain, Shakti. *Creative Visualization*. New York: Bantam, 1982.

Hammitzsch, Horst. *Zen in the Art of the Tea Ceremony*. New York: Penguin, 1993.

Hanh, Thich Nhat. *The Miracle of Mindfulness*. Boston: Beacon Press, 1975.

Ind, Joe. *Fat Is a Spiritual Issue: My Journey*. New York: Mowbray, 1993.

Kabat-Zinn, Jon. *Full Catastrophe Living*. New York: Delacorte Press, 1990.

Kalechofsky, Roberta, ed. *Rabbis and Vegetarianism: An Evolving Tradition*. Marblehead, MA: Micah Publications, Inc., 1995.

Kaplan, Aryeh. *Jewish Meditation: A Practical Guide*. New York: Schocken Books, 1985.

Kesten, Deborah. *Feeding the Body, Nourishing the Soul*. Berkeley, CA: Conari Press, 1998.

Kornfield, Jack. *Living Dharma: Teachings of Twelve Buddhist Masters*. Boston: Shambhala, 1996.

Lasher, Margot. *The Art and Practice of Compassion*. New York: Tarcher/Putnam, 1992.

Laskow, Leonard. *Healing with Love: A Breakthrough Mind/Body Medical Program for Healing Yourself and Others*. San Francisco: HarperCollins, 1992.

Loori, Abbot John Daido. *Master Dogen's Metaphysics of Eating*. Mt. Tremper, NY: Dharma Communications, 1994; audiocassette.

Madison, Deborah, with Edward Espe Brown. *The Greens Cookbook: Extraordinary Vegetarian Cuisine from the Celebrated Restaurant*. Toronto and New York: Bantam, 1987.

McEachern, Alton H. *Here at Thy Table Lord: Enriching the Observance of the Lord's Supper*. Nashville, TN: Broadman Press, 1977.

McGee, Charles T., with Effie Poy Yew Chow. *QiGong: Miracle Healing from China*. Cour d'Alene, ID: MediPress, 1996.

Okakura, Kakuzo. *The Book of Tea*. Boston and London: Shambhala, 1993.

Ornish, Dean. *Dr. Dean Ornish's Program for Reversing Heart Disease*. New York: Random House, 1990.

_____. *Eat More, Weigh Less*. New York: HarperCollins, 1993.

_____. *Love and Survival: The Scientific Basis for the Healing Power of Intimacy*. New York: HarperCollins, 1998.

Pert, Candace. *Molecules of Emotion: Why You Feel the Way You Feel*. New York: Scribner, 1997.

Rain, Mary Summer. *Ancient Echoes: The Anasazi Book of Chants*. Norfolk, VA: Hampton Roads, 1993.

Remen, Rachel Naomi. *Kitchen Table Wisdom*. New York: Riverhead Books, 1996.

Rubik, Beverly. *Life at the Edge of Science*. Philadelphia, PA: The Institute for Frontier Science, 1996.

Sakr, Ahmad H. *Dietary Regulations and Food Habits of Muslims*. New York: Muslim World League, 1976.

Scherwitz, Larry, et al. "Self-involvement and Coronary Heart Disease Incidence in the Multiple Risk Factor Intervention Trial." *Psychosomatic Medicine* 48 (1986): 187–99.

_____. "Self-Involvement and the Risk Factors for Coronary Heart Disease." *Advances* 2 (1985): 6–18.

Sen, Soshitsu, XV. *The Urasenke Tradition of Tea*. Kyoto, Japan: Urasenke Foundation, 1983.

Shaffer, Carolyn, and Kristin Anundsen. *Creating Community Anywhere*. New York: Tarcher/Putnam, 1993.

Shendelman, Sara, and Avram Davis. *Traditions: The Complete*

Book of Prayers, Rituals, and Blessings for Every Jewish Home. New York: Hyperion, 1998.

Smith, Huston. *The Illustrated World's Religions: A Guide to Our Wisdom Traditions.* San Francisco: HarperCollins, 1994.

Somer, Elizabeth. *Food and Mood: The Complete Guide to Feeling Well and Eating Your Best.* New York: Holt, 1994.

Stacy, Michelle. *Consumed: Why Americans Love, Hate, and Fear Food.* New York: Touchstone, 1994.

Sterling, Richard, ed. *Food: True Stories of Life on the Road.* San Francisco, CA: Travelers' Tales, 1996.

Tompkins, Peter, and Christopher Bird. *The Secret Life of Plants.* New York: Harper & Row, 1973.

Wilbur, Ken. *The Spectrum of Consciousness.* Wheaton, IL: Quest Books, 1993.

Wolf, Burt. *Gatherings and Celebrations: History, Folklore, Rituals and Recipes for the Occasions That Bring People Together.* New York: Doubleday, 1996.

Wurtman, Judith J. *Managing Your Mind and Mood Through Food.* New York: Rawson Associates, 1986.

Zohar, Danah. *The Quantum Self: Human Nature and Consciousness Defined by the New Physics.* New York: Quill, 1990.

index

F

G

about the author

Originally from New York City, Deborah Kesten, M.P.H., developed an expertise in nutrition while obtaining a master's degree in public health from the University of Texas School of Public Health and a bachelor's in the health sciences from the University of Houston, where she graduated magna cum laude. She began her career as the nutrition educator with physician and best-selling author Dean Ornish, M.D., on his first clinical trial for reversing heart disease.

A pioneer in the field on nutritional science, Kesten has participated in lifestyle and nutrition research in the United States and Europe, and has lectured in India over the past fifteen years. Her work as a researcher, lecturer, and health journalist has established her as an international leader in integrative nutrition.

Ms. Kesten has authored more than eighty articles in national and international journals and magazines, including the *Journal of the American Medical Association, Yoga Journal,* and *Veggie Life.* Her first book, *Feeding the Body, Nourishing the Soul,* received the prestigious Independent Publishers' Book Award in 1998, and she was honored as a "healer for the new millennium" by Healthy Living magazine. She has taught courses on integrative nutrition at California Pacific Medical Center's Institute for Health and Healing in San Francisco, lectured at San Francisco State University's Department of Holistic Health, and continues to lecture and conduct workshops internationally. Ms. Kesten lives in Sausalito, California, with her husband, Larry Scherwitz, Ph.D.

Lucky Vitamin
Vitacost
DRS BEST Celadrin
500 mg / 90 caps
joint mobility

New World Library is dedicated to
publishing books and cassettes that inspire
and challenge us to improve the quality
of our lives and our world.
Our books and cassettes are available
at bookstores everywhere.
For a complete catalog, contact:

New World Library
14 Pamaron Way
Novato, California 94949
Phone: (415) 884-2100
Fax: (415) 884-2199
Or call toll free: (800) 972-6657
Catalog requests: Ext. 50
Ordering: Ext. 52
E-mail: escort@nwlib.com
newworldlibrary.com